JN246958

English for Healthcare Communication

すぐに使える医療・看護英語

Mami Inoue

Rieko Matsuoka

Ruri Ashida

Tamiko Miyatsu

Jeffrey Huffman

MEDICAL VIEW

English for Healthcare Communication

(ISBN978-4-7583-0759-8 C3047)

Authors : Mami Inoue, Rieko Matsuoka, Ruri Ashida, Tamiko Miyatsu,
 Jeffrey Huffman

2016. 1.10 1st ed.

©MEDICAL VIEW, 2016
Printed and Bound in Japan

Medical View Co., Ltd.
2-30 Ichigaya-honmuracho, Shinjuku-ku, Tokyo, 162-0845, Japan
E-mail ed@medicalview.co.jp

はじめに

　グローバル化に伴い，日本においても医療の国際化が急速に進み，医療・看護に特化した英語コミュニケーション能力の必要性が高まっています。実際，今後ますます日本で受診する外国人の患者さんが増え，医療従事者には優れた医療技術と共に実践的なコミュニケーション能力が必要とされるでしょう。

　本書は，関東の医療・看護学関連の英語教育に携わる教員が2013年にネットワークを形成し，協力して立ち上げたプロジェクト（仮称 Japan Association of Nursing English Education［JANEE］／プロジェクト本部 聖路加国際大学）のワーキンググループが開発した看護学生のための英語テキストです。プロジェクトでは，グローバル化が進む医療・看護の分野の英語教育に有効な教科書とはどういうものであるかを話し合ってきました。プロジェクトメンバーの先生方との発展的な意見交換を通して生まれたのが本書です。具体的には，医療の国際化に対応できる人材（nursing professionals with transcultural competence）の養成を目指し，国際化した日本の医療現場で看護師に求められる①実践的な英語コミュニケーション能力の養成，②異文化コミュニケーションに必要な知識の獲得の2点に焦点を絞りました。

　テキストは「患者ケア」，「成育ケア」，「慢性病ケア」，「入退院ケア」の4つのユニットで構成されています。各ユニットは3つのレッスンから成り，それぞれテーマに沿った医療シーンを想定し，そのシーンでのダイアローグを中心として以下の通り展開します。

I　Reading and Discussion

II　Post-Reading Vocabulary

III　Pre-Listening Vocabulary

IV　Extra Vocabulary

V　Listening (Dialog・Key Expressions) / Cross-Cultural Topics

VI　Communication Activity

　特に，さまざまな場面設定でのダイアローグとそれらを用いたCommunication Activityは，医療シーンでの基礎的な会話表現だけでなく，わかりやすく丁寧な説明や指導，共感の示し方など，外国人の患者さんに接する際に大切な表現方法が習得できるよう工夫されています。医療職を目指す学生が本書での学びを基礎として，実践的なコミュニケーション能力と異文化間能力を伸ばし，将来，国内外で活躍してくれることを期待しています。

2015年12月

著者一同

目次 Table of Contents

Extra Vocabulary	Cross-Cultural Topics	Communication Activity
Body Parts	アメリカの医療制度について Health Insurance System in the US	初診患者に対応する First Visit Examination
Supplies and Equipment	世界救急車事情 Ambulance Services around the World	痛みをアセスメントをする Pain Assessment
Digestive System	人間ドックを説明できますか A Full Physical Exam Called 'Human Dock'	検査を説明する Instructions for Medical Tests

Appendix: Departments and Specialists (p. 26)

Extra Vocabulary	Cross-Cultural Topics	Communication Activity
Reproductive Organs	ウィメンズヘルスと異文化理解 OB/GYN Cultural Considerations	婦人科の診療の説明をする Explaining a Gynecological Examination
Stages of Labor	女性と家族の健やかな人生を支える助産師 Midwifery around the World	離乳食指導をする Offering Weaning Advice
Vaccination	相手の立場に立った コミュニケーション Cultural Competence in Clinical Communication	予防接種の説明をする Explaining Vaccinations

Appendix: Doctors, Nurses, Allied Health Professionals (p. 52)

	Pages	Post-Reading Vocabulary	Pre-Listening Vocabulary	
Unit 3 **Chronic Illness** 慢性病ケア	53 〜 78			
Lesson 1 **Lifestyle-Related Disease**	54 〜 61	· angina pectoris · palpitations · chronic disease · obese	· lifestyle-related disease · consulting room · bypass surgery · diet	
Lesson 2 **Dietary Restrictions**	62 〜 69	· dietary restrictions · dialysis · kidney failure · non-adherence	· underweight · confusion · low-sodium diet · shortness of breath	
Lesson 3 **Dementia**	70 〜 77	· dementia · depression · mild cognitive impairment · personality change	· memory loss · irritated · wandering · moody	

	Pages	Post-Reading Vocabulary	Pre-Listening Vocabulary	
Unit 4 **Inpatient Care** 入退院ケア	79 〜 104			
Lesson 1 **Admission for Surgery**	80 〜 87	· gallstones · laparoscopic surgery · guarantor · admission	· informed consent · urinary catheter · painkiller · inpatient	
Lesson 2 **Daily Life in the Hospital**	88 〜 95	· vital signs · ward · tonsils · postoperative	· urination · bowel movement · bed bath · visiting hours	
Lesson 3 **Discharge and Home Care**	96 〜 103	· chest tube · discharge · wound care · oral chemotherapy	· drowsiness · general practitioner (GP) · home care · caregiver	

Extra Vocabulary	Cross-Cultural Topics	Communication Activity
Circulatory System	行列大国ニッポン "I've been waiting for a long time!"	院内の案内をする Giving Directions
Excretory System	世界の臓器移植事情 Organ Transplantation around the World	食事制限についてたずねる Asking about Dietary Restrictions
Aids for the Elderly	終の棲家はどこ？ Where is Your Final Home?	患者の家族を支援する Supporting the Patient's Family
Appendix: Diseases (p. 78)		
Surgery	入院から退院、そして在宅医療へ From Hospitalization to Home Care	手術と入院の説明をする Giving Information about Surgery and Hospitalization
Bedside	入院生活を支えるケア Supporting Patients' Daily Life in the Hospital	入院中の生活を補助する Helping Patients during Their Hospital Stay
Respiratory System	一人ひとりの最期の時 A Person's Last Moment	退院指導をする Giving Discharge Instructions
Appendix: Measurements and Tests (p. 104)		
Glossary (p. 105 〜 107)		

●著者
井上麻未（聖路加国際大学）
松岡里枝子（国立看護大学校）
芦田ルリ（東京慈恵会医科大学）
宮津多美子（順天堂大学）
Jeffrey Huffman（聖路加国際大学）

●医事監修
中村 正（なかむら ただし）
なかむら耳鼻咽喉科クリニック院長
元 山形大学医学部准教授
同臨床教授
英国 National Hospital for Neurology and Neurosurgery 研究員
現 聖マリアンナ医科大学非常勤講師

Jan Opdahl（オプダール ジャン）
元 米国ボカラトンコミュニティ病院　正看護師
元 米国聖ヨセフ病院　トラベルナース
元 西町インターナショナルスクール　スクールナース
聖路加国際大学 非常勤講師

〈表紙イラスト〉
羽馬有紗

〈写真提供（50 音順）〉
アズワン株式会社
アルケア株式会社
株式会社バイテック・グローバル・ジャパン
株式会社フタバ
サラヤ株式会社
東芝メディカルシステムズ（株）
パナソニック エイジフリーライフテック（株）
フランスベッド株式会社
リオン株式会社

■音声ダウンロード方法
①本書リスニング問題は，音声をダウンロードすることが可能です。
②下記 URL にアクセスしてください。

　http://www.medicalview.co.jp/download/ISBN978-4-7583-0759-8/

③本書の音声再生ページが表示されますので，利用規約に同意の上，ご利用ください。「音声を聴く」ボタンをクリックすると音声が再生されます。ダウンロードする場合はご使用のブラウザのヘルプをご覧ください。
注）お使いの PC・スマートフォン・タブレット端末の種類やブラウザによっては正常に再生・ダウンロードできない場合があります。

本書の解答集をご希望の方にお分けいたします（ただし，授業の教材として利用されている学生の方は除きます）。ご希望の方は必ず書面（FAX，E-mail も可）にて，氏名・勤務先・送付先住所を明記のうえ，下記へお申し込みください。

申し込み先：メジカルビュー社 編集部 医学英語書籍担当者
〒 162-0845　東京都新宿区市谷本村町 2-30
FAX 0120-77-2062
E-mail ed@medicalview.co.jp

Unit 1　患者ケア

Outpatient Care

　このユニットでは，外来病棟における外国人患者さんへの対応やケアについて学びます。日程が限られている出張や観光旅行で訪れた旅先での病気やケガは予期せぬ結果を招きます。もし日本に滞在する外国人の方がこのような状況に陥ったとき，皆さんは医療者従事者としてどのように対応すればよいのでしょうか。また，今後ますます需要が増えていくと考えられる医療ツーリズムの患者さんに対して，医療者として気を付けることはどんなことでしょうか。

　ここでは，感染性疾患のインフルエンザ，観光地でのケガによる救急外来，医療ツーリズム（もしくは医療観光）の事例を扱います。課題を通して異文化理解に必要なことは何なのか学びましょう。

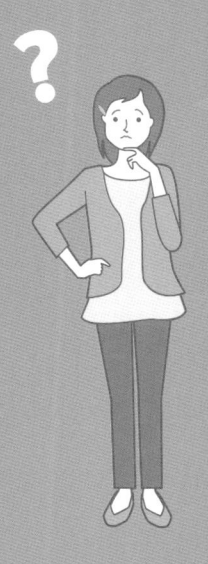

考えてみよう

Q1　来日外国人数が最も多いのは，
アジア，北米，ヨーロッパ，どの地域？

Q2　短期滞在をする外国人の来日目的で多いのは
観光？ 商用？

Q3　医療ツーリズムの定義は？

Visit to the Clinic

I Reading and Discussion

以下の文章を読んで患者情報を完成させなさい。また，1 ～ 3 の質問に英語で答えなさい。

Mary Baker, a 46-year-old American bank executive, is visiting Japan to make a presentation at an important meeting. Despite her busy schedule, she has found time to visit Sensoji Temple, Yanaka Ginza, and the Imperial Palace. However, she has been suffering from a very sore throat for three days now, so she came to Dr. Aoki's clinic in Harajuku. She has also been feeling feverish since last night. Her other symptoms include a bad cough and joint pain, and she has lost her appetite completely. The coughing has been keeping her awake throughout the night. Her flight leaves for New York tomorrow. Will she be able to board the plane, or will she have to postpone her flight? A nurse at the clinic is attending to Ms. Baker. She starts by asking Ms. Baker to fill out a questionnaire.

Patient Information

Name: _____ Nationality: _____

Age: _____ Occupation: _____

Gender: _____ Chief Concerns: _____

1 **Why did Ms. Baker come to Japan?**

2 **Did Ms. Baker have a good sleep last night? Why or why not?**

3 **What questions do you think the nurse will ask Ms. Baker?**

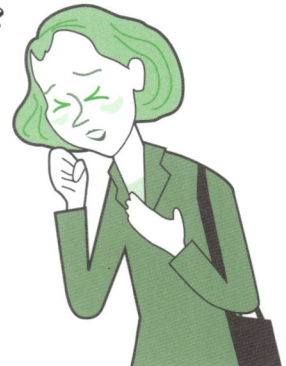

Ⅱ Post-Reading Vocabulary

空欄に入る語をボックスから選び，記号で答えなさい。

1 When a child is (　　　　　), an American parent would bathe her/him in lukewarm water.

2 Do you have any other (　　　　　) besides your cough?

3 A (　　　　　) may make it difficult to speak or swallow food.

4 The old man had trouble using stairs because of the (　　　　　) in his knees.

> **ⓐ** sore throat　　**ⓑ** feverish　　**ⓒ** symptoms　　**ⓓ** joint pain

Ⅲ Pre-Listening Vocabulary

以下の語の定義をボックスから選び，記号で答えなさい。

1 questionnaire　(　　　　　)

2 chills　　　　(　　　　　)

3 appetite　　　(　　　　　)

4 specimen　　　(　　　　　)

> **ⓐ** the feeling of being hungry
> **ⓑ** feeling cold
> **ⓒ** a small amount of tissue or fluid taken from the body
> **ⓓ** a written list of questions for collecting necessary information

Ⅳ Extra Vocabulary (Body Parts)

イラストに対応する語をボックスから選び，記号で答えなさい。

1 （　　　　）
2 （　　　　）
3 （　　　　）
4 （　　　　）
5 （　　　　）
6 （　　　　）
7 （　　　　）
8 （　　　　）
9 （　　　　）
10 （　　　　）
11 （　　　　）

12 （　　　　）
13 （　　　　）
14 （　　　　）
15 （　　　　）
16 （　　　　）
17 （　　　　）
18 （　　　　）

19 （　　　　）
20 （　　　　）
21 （　　　　）
22 （　　　　）
23 （　　　　）
24 （　　　　）
25 （　　　　）
26 （　　　　）

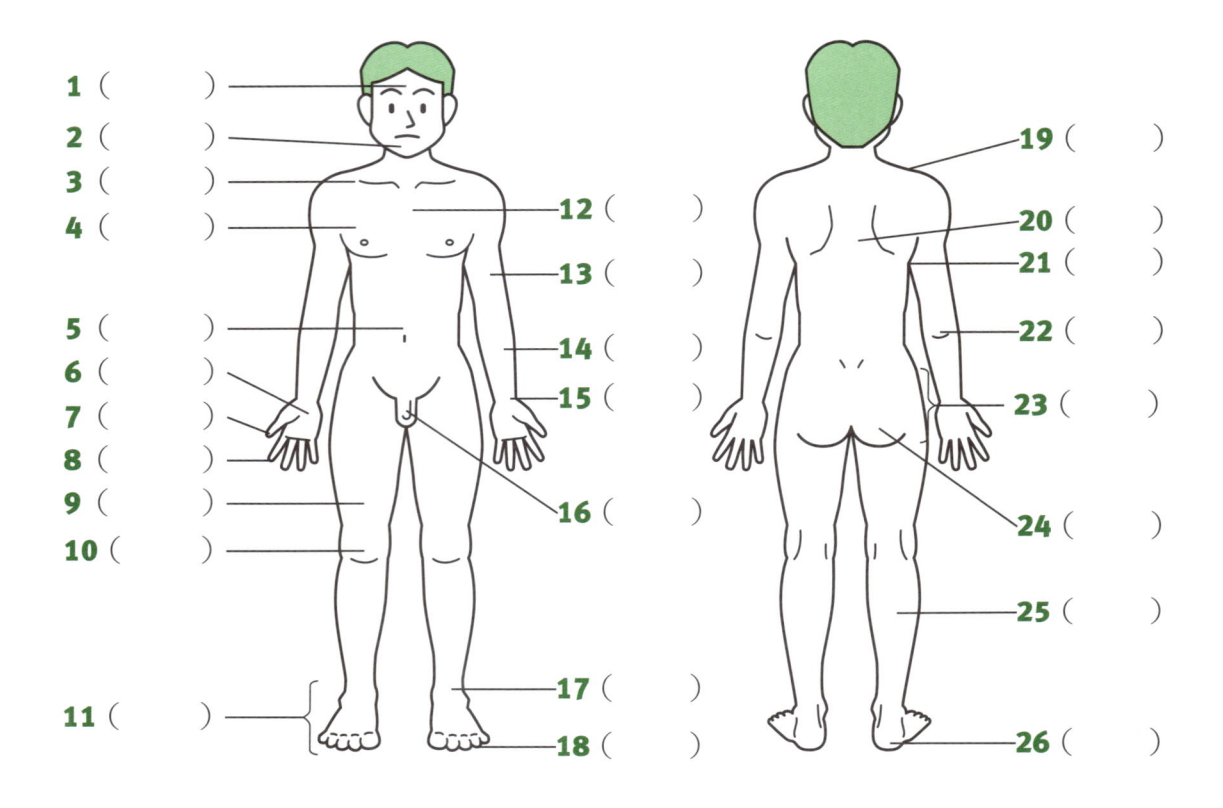

ⓐ heel	**ⓑ** chest	**ⓒ** abdomen	**ⓓ** hip	**ⓔ** forehead
ⓕ elbow	**ⓖ** breast	**ⓗ** genitals	**ⓘ** calf	**ⓙ** back
ⓚ clavicle (collarbone)		**ⓛ** toe	**ⓜ** axilla (armpit)	**ⓝ** palm
ⓞ jaw	**ⓟ** knee	**ⓠ** forearm	**ⓡ** buttocks (bottom)	
ⓢ thumb	**ⓣ** ankle	**ⓤ** finger	**ⓥ** shoulder	**ⓦ** foot
ⓧ thigh	**ⓨ** wrist	**ⓩ** upper arm		

Ⅴ Listening

AUDIO 1-1

看護師と患者さんの会話を聞いて，以下の質問の答えとして最も適当なものを選びなさい。

1 Who is going to fill out the questionnaire? Why?
- **a** Ms. Baker will, because the nurse asked her to do it.
- **b** The nurse will, because Ms. Baker cannot read Japanese.
- **c** Ms. Baker will, because the questionnaire is in English.
- **d** The nurse will, because Ms. Baker's hands hurt.

2 Which is NOT one of Ms. Baker's symptoms?
- **a** fever
- **b** sore throat
- **c** joint pain
- **d** chest pain

3 Why does the doctor use a cotton swab?
- **a** to take a specimen from Ms. Baker's nose
- **b** to hold Ms. Baker's mouth open
- **c** to look inside Ms. Baker's throat
- **d** to look inside Ms. Baker's nose

4 Why can't Ms. Baker fly home tomorrow?
- **a** She is too weak.
- **b** She has one more meeting in Tokyo.
- **c** She cannot get on the plane while she has the flu.
- **d** Her flight was cancelled.

5 Why does Ms. Baker have to pay the full cost?
- **a** She is in Tokyo on business.
- **b** She doesn't have insurance.
- **c** She forgot to bring her insurance card.
- **d** She only has traveler's insurance.

Dialog

Ms. Baker	Excuse me. Can you speak English?
Nurse	Yes, a little. What brings you here today?
Ms. Baker	I have a sore throat and a bad cough.
Nurse	I see. Okay, would you mind filling out this questionnaire?
Ms. Baker	Oh… well, I can't read Japanese… and I'm feeling really sick. Could you fill it out for me?
Nurse	Sure. OK, can you describe your symptoms for me?
Ms. Baker	Well, as I said, I have a sore throat and a bad cough. And I feel feverish and have chills, and I have some joint pain, too. And I've completely lost my appetite.
Nurse	Well, these seem like typical flu symptoms, so the doctor will probably use a cotton swab to take a specimen from your nose. It might feel a bit uncomfortable.
	[*Later*]
Nurse	Ms. Baker, as the doctor said, the test showed that you have type A influenza. Be sure to take the medicine, get plenty of rest, and drink lots of fluids. Do you have any other questions?
Ms. Baker	I'm worried about my flight tomorrow. Do you think I'll be able to fly back to New York?
Nurse	Oh no, unfortunately that will be impossible. Even if you feel strong enough, you will not be allowed to board the plane if you have the flu.
Ms. Baker	I was also wondering about the payment. I have traveler's insurance that should cover it.
Receptionist	OK, but I'm afraid you will have to pay the full cost now, and then you can get reimbursed by your insurance company later.

Key Expressions

1 What brings you here today?
今日はどうなさったのですか。

2 Would you mind filling out this questionnaire?
問診票にご記入いただいてもよろしいですか。

3 Can you describe your symptoms for me?
どんな症状があるか説明していただけますか。

4 It might feel a bit uncomfortable.
少し不快に感じるかもしれません。

5 Be sure to take the medicine, get plenty of rest, and drink lots of fluids.
薬を飲み，十分に休息し，水分を多くとるようにしてください。

Cross-Cultural Topics

アメリカの医療制度について　Health Insurance System in the US

　国民皆保険の国に生きる私たちには奇異に感じますが，イギリスなど国営保険制度（NHS）を有し，無料で医療サービスを受けることが可能な国がある一方で，アメリカには日本の国民健康保険制度にあたる制度はありません。自由診療のアメリカでの医療費は高額です。アメリカ滞在中，急性咽頭炎に罹って1日入院した際，約2,700ドルも請求されてショックを受けたという方もいます。

　アメリカでは，連邦政府の医療プログラムとして，高齢者および障害者向けの公的医療保険であるメディケア（Medicare），低所得者に対する公的医療保険制度であるメディケイド（Medicaid）の2種類がありますが，これとは別に，多くの人は独自に主に民間の医療保険に加入することでより質の高い医療サービスを受けています。2014年，全国民の医療保険の加入促進を目的とする医療保険制度改革法（Patient Protection and Affordable Care Act：通称オバマケア）が施行され，メディケアへの加入資格は拡大されましたが，立案・運営は州の裁量に任されているため，これによって提供される医療サービスは決して均一とはいえません（メディケア支出は州と連邦政府で折半）。財政的理由から医療提供者への支払額を減額した州では，赤字を恐れた病院や医師がメディケイド患者の診察を拒否するといった事態も起こっています。今後，「オバマケア」で無保険者の数は減ってゆくと予想されますが，増え続ける医療費により，制度自体が破たんする恐れも指摘されています。アメリカの医療保険制度改革は今後どのように進んでいくのでしょう。

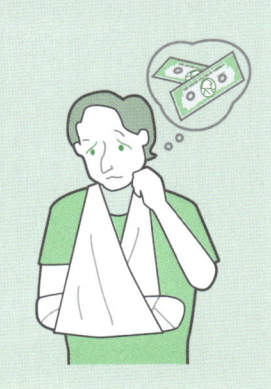

Communication Activity
初診患者に対応する First Visit Examination

看護師役と患者さん役に分かれて，以下のモデルダイアローグを練習しましょう。

Example Scenario: Ali Fadavi is an Iranian painter. He lives in Tokyo now. He had chills early in the morning and noticed he was feverish. So he visited the clinic.

STEP 1

Model dialog

Nurse	So Mr. Fadavi, you have chills and feel feverish, right?
Mr. Fadavi	Correct, it started early this morning.
Nurse	OK, let me take your temperature. Please put this thermometer in your armpit.
Mr. Fadavi	All right. [*beeping*]
Nurse	Oh, it's 38.5 degrees Celsius, which is a bit higher than 101 degrees Fahrenheit. Please wait here. The doctor will see you soon.
Mr. Fadavi	Thanks.

ボックスの中の表現を使って，以下の会話を練習しましょう。

Scenario 1: Mary Davis comes to see a doctor with her son, David. He has a runny nose and a terrible cough. The nurse asks her to fill out the questionnaire first and then asks about her son's symptoms. The nurse then directs them to an examination room.

STEP 2

Nurse	① _____
Ms. Davis	Well, as you can see, my son David has a runny nose and he's coughing a lot.
Nurse	② _____ ③ _____
Ms. Davis	All right. [*beeping*] Here you are.
Nurse	④ _____ Please wait here, and the doctor will see you soon.

> ⓐ Hello, what brings you here today?
>
> ⓑ Thanks. He is a bit feverish.
>
> ⓒ Please put this thermometer in his armpit.
>
> ⓓ OK, let's take his temperature.

以下の手順に従って，会話の練習をしましょう。

Scenario 2: Alex Burns is a university student studying Japanese history. After working all night on his class paper, he started to feel nauseated and he vomited. So he is now at the clinic near his school.

Procedure

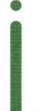

❶ Greet the patient.

❷ Ask him/her to fill out the questionnaire.

❸ Confirm what the problem is.

❹ Tell the patient what to do.

Medical Information Sheet

Name		☐ Male ☐ Female
Address		Date of birth (DOB)
Phone number		
Nationality	Religion	
Marital status	Occupation	
Do you have health insurance?	☐ Yes	☐ No

What are your symptoms?

fever	headache	stomachache	runny nose
dizziness	nausea	coughing	itching
rash	constipation	diarrhea	

Pain (Where? _____) Others (_____)

What is your main concern?

How long have you had these symptoms?

Are you currently taking medication?   ☐ Yes ☐ No

If yes, what kind is it? _____

Have you had any serious illness or diseases in the past?   ☐ Yes ☐ No

If yes, what was it? _____

Have you ever had surgery?   ☐ Yes ☐ No

If yes, what for? _____

Unit 1

Lesson 2

Injury and Pain

I Reading and Discussion

以下の文章を読んで患者情報を完成させなさい。また、1〜3の質問に英語で答えなさい。

John and Emma Evans from England are a young married couple. Mr. Evans is 27 years old and Mrs. Evans is 25 years old. They are visiting Japan for their honeymoon because Mrs. Evans majored in East Asian Studies at a university in the UK. She wanted to take this opportunity to experience Japanese culture firsthand. Mr. Evans, who is a chef, is interested in Japanese cuisine, which has become popular in the UK. After enjoying the Kyoto area, they visited Yokohama. Unfortunately, Mr. Evans fell down the stairs at a temple. He could not walk because of the sharp pain in his left ankle. Mrs. Evans asked the monk to call an ambulance. The ambulance arrived and he was brought to the ER at the nearest hospital.

Patient Information

Name: _____

Nationality: _____

Age: _____

Occupation: _____

Gender: _____

Chief Concerns: _____

1 Why are Mr. and Mrs. Evans in Japan?

2 Where did they visit?

3 What do you think the ER nurse will ask Mr. Evans?

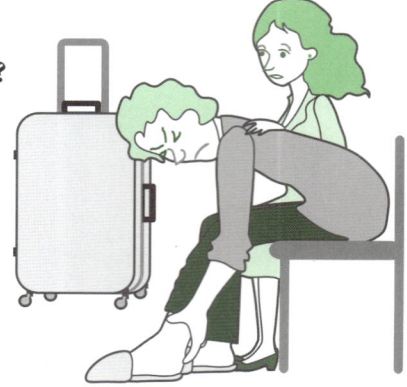

Ⅱ Post-Reading Vocabulary

空欄に入る語をボックスから選び，記号で答えなさい。

1 The injured man was taken to the hospital by ( ).

2 If you ( ) your ankle, it will be painful to walk.

3 In order to find out if my toe was broken, I had an ( ) taken.

4 If you call 119, you will be taken to the ( ).

ⓐ ER	**ⓑ** ambulance	**ⓒ** X-ray	**ⓓ** sprain

Ⅲ Pre-Listening Vocabulary

以下の語の定義をボックスから選び，記号で答えなさい。

1 breath ( )

2 heal ( )

3 fracture ( )

4 prescribe ( )

ⓐ to become healthy or feel better
ⓑ a break in a bone or other hard material
ⓒ to write an order for medicine for a patient
ⓓ the air that we take into our lungs and send out

Ⅳ Extra Vocabulary (Supplies and Equipment)

写真に対応する語をボックスから選び，記号で答えなさい。

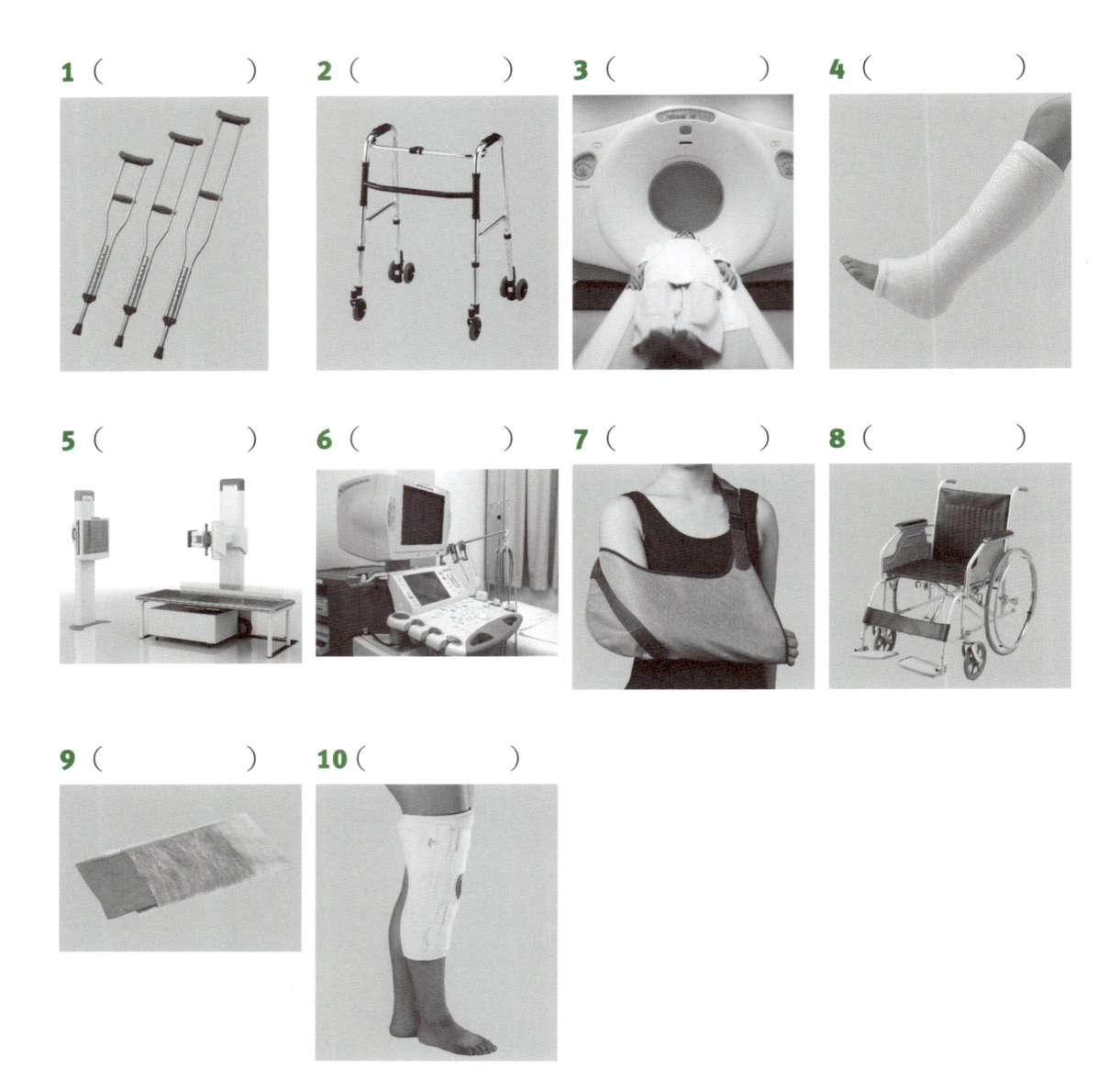

1 (　　　　　)　2 (　　　　　)　3 (　　　　　)　4 (　　　　　)

5 (　　　　　)　6 (　　　　　)　7 (　　　　　)　8 (　　　　　)

9 (　　　　　)　10 (　　　　　)

- ⓐ CT scanner
- ⓑ ultrasound machine
- ⓒ X-ray machine
- ⓓ cast
- ⓔ crutches
- ⓕ sling
- ⓖ walker
- ⓗ wheelchair
- ⓘ cold compress/pack
- ⓙ supporter

Ⅴ Listening

AUDIO 1-2

看護師と患者さんの会話を聞いて，以下の質問の答えとして最も適切なものを選びなさい。

1 How was Mr. Evans injured?
ⓐ He was in a bicycle accident.
ⓑ He fell down some stairs.
ⓒ Someone stepped on his foot.
ⓓ He dropped a heavy box on his foot.

2 What was the cause of his pain?
ⓐ He fractured his leg.
ⓑ He scraped his knee.
ⓒ He sprained his ankle.
ⓓ He bumped his toe.

3 Does he have to be hospitalized?
ⓐ Yes, he has to stay in the hospital overnight.
ⓑ Yes, but there is no room available.
ⓒ No, he does not need to stay overnight.
ⓓ No, he cannot be hospitalized because he has no insurance.

4 What kind of test did he have?
ⓐ blood test
ⓑ urinalysis
ⓒ ultrasound
ⓓ X-ray

5 Does Mr. Evans need to see the doctor again?
ⓐ Yes, the next day.
ⓑ Yes, in one week.
ⓒ Only if the terrible pain continues.
ⓓ No, he does not.

Dialog

Nurse   Are you all right? You are at the hospital now. We're going to take good care of you. Can you tell me what happened to you?

Mr. Evans   Well, I slipped and fell down the stairs at a temple. I have a sharp pain in my ankle and cannot walk.

Nurse   Which ankle is it?

Mr. Evans   [*groaning*] The left one. I'm in terrible pain!

Nurse   I see. Try to take some deep breaths. The doctor will see you as soon as possible.

[The doctor examines Mr. Evans and then asks the nurse to take him to get an X-ray.]

Nurse   I'm going to take you to the X-ray Department now.

[After the X-ray, the nurse wheels Mr. Evans back to the examination room.]

Doctor   Please come in. [*He examines the X-ray film.*] Can you see this here? Your ankle is not fractured—it's only sprained. You are lucky.

Mr. Evans   Yeah, I can see it. I'm so glad it's not broken. My wife Emma and I are here for our honeymoon. Will I need to stay in the hospital?

Doctor   No, that won't be necessary. I will prescribe some pain medicine for you.

Mr. Evans   Yes, I'm sure I'll need that!

Nurse   You'll also need to use these crutches for a few days. I hope your ankle heals fast. Please call us if you have any problem.

Mr. Evans   OK. Thanks so much for all of your assistance.

Key Expressions

1 We are going to take good care of you.
十分にお世話させていただきますね。

2 Can you tell me what happened to you?
どうなさったのか教えてくださいますか。

3 Try to take some deep breaths.
何回が深呼吸をなさってみてください。

4 I am going to take you to the X-ray Department now.
これから放射線科にお連れします。

5 Please call us if you have any problem.
何かございましたら，こちらにお電話してください。

Cross-Cultural Topics

世界救急車事情　Ambulance Services around the World

　日本では119番で救急車を呼べば，迅速に病院まで救急搬送してくれます。私たち市民誰もが安心して利用できる救急車ですが，救急車の出動件数は一貫して増加傾向にあり，現場までの到着時間が年々遅くなっているという現状があります（総務省消防庁 消防白書）。さらに，救急車で搬送される人の約半数は軽症者であるため，不要不急の出動により緊急を要する重症者への対応が遅れるという問題点も指摘されています。日本の救急車は無料ですが，海外の多くの国では救急車は有料です。アメリカ，フランス，ドイツなどでは救急出動だけで数万円が必要です（外務省 世界の医療事情）。中国では救急車は「救護（護）車」といい，有料でしかも前払いです。韓国

では無料ですが，民間の有料のものもあります。イギリスは日本と同様に救急車は無料ですが，日本に比べて病院での待ち時間が長く，命に関わる症状ではない場合には対応は迅速ではありません。救急車を安心して利用できる日本の医療システムを今後も維持してゆくためには，救急車は緊急を要する人が利用するものという当たり前のことを再確認する必要があるでしょう。

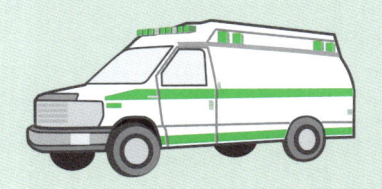

Communication Activity
痛みをアセスメントする（ペインスケール参照）Pain Assessment

STEP 1

看護師役と患者さん役に分かれて，以下のモデルダイアローグを練習しましょう。

Example Scenario: Emily Whitaker twisted her ankle two days ago while riding her bike, and it is very painful. It is a throbbing pain. She thought the pain would go away soon, but instead it became stronger, so she visited the clinic.

Model dialog

Nurse	Are you all right? You look like you are in pain.
Ms. Whitaker	Oh, yes, my ankle hurts intensely.
Nurse	Can you tell me what happened?
Ms. Whitaker	Well, I twisted my ankle two days ago while cycling.
Nurse	Oh, two days ago?
Ms. Whitaker	That's right. Actually, I thought the pain would go away, but it has become worse.
Nurse	Which ankle is it? Please show me exactly where it hurts.
Ms. Whitaker	It's my left ankle, and it hurts right here.
Nurse	How painful is it, based on this chart?
Ms. Whitaker	I think 6 or 7.
Nurse	All right. The doctor will see you soon.

STEP 2

ボックスの中の表現を使って，以下の会話を練習しましょう。

Scenario 1: Lucy Vickers is a homemaker whose husband works for a Japanese trading company. She has lived in Japan for a few years, and has enjoyed cooking Japanese dishes. One day she burned her hand when cooking tempura. She is now at a clinic near her condominium.

Nurse	Are you all right? You look like you are in great pain.
Ms. Vickers	Yes, look at this. This is really nasty.
Nurse	① _____
Ms. Vickers	OK. Yesterday, when I was cooking tempura, I burned my hand with oil.
Nurse	② _____
Ms. Vickers	Yes, I tried to cool the burns with running water.
Nurse	③ _____
Ms. Vickers	Do you think I will have scars?
Nurse	④ _____
Ms. Vickers	All right.

ⓐ I'm not sure. You can ask the doctor later, though.

ⓑ Did you cool your burns?

ⓒ Can you tell me what happened?

ⓓ You did what you are supposed to do.

STEP 3

以下の手順に従って，会話の練習をしましょう。

Scenario 2: Mariam Robertson has been suffering from severe pain in her neck as a result of whiplash. She was bumped from behind when she was driving a month ago, and has been undergoing physiotherapy since then. However, she still has pain in the evening. She decides to visit an orthopedic clinic which her good friend recommended.

Procedure

❶ Ask about what happened.

❷ Assess the type of pain and the location.

❸ Ask when the pain started.

❹ Use the pain scale to ask how severe the pain is.

❺ Tell the patient to wait until the doctor is ready to see her.

Pain Terminology

1 *What kind of pain it is?*

dull	sharp	throbbing	crampy	burning
piercing/stabbing	mild	constant	intermittent (comes and goes)	

2 *Where does it hurt?*

throat   neck   chest   stomach   ankle   back

3 *How severe is the pain?*

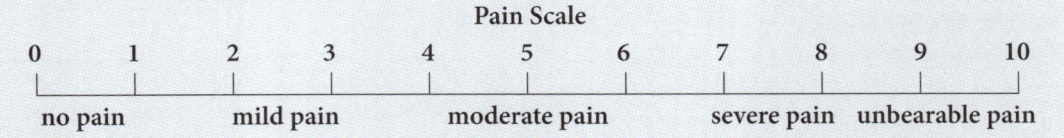

Pain Scale

0	1	2	3	4	5	6	7	8	9	10

no pain   mild pain   moderate pain   severe pain   unbearable pain

4 *When did the pain start? How long have you had the pain?*

since yesterday   a couple of days ago   for three days

Other Useful Expressions

1. Can you tell me what happened to you?
2. What kind of pain do you have? Where does it hurt?
3. When did the pain start?
4. What level is your pain on this scale?
5. Look at this scale. Please tell me how painful you feel.
6. You will have an MRI in order to find the problem.
7. Could you wait in the waiting room for a while? We will call you when the doctor is ready.

Medical Examination

I Reading and Discussion

以下の文章を読んで患者情報を完成させなさい。また，1 〜 3 の質問に英語で答えなさい。

Ivan Antonov, who is an airplane pilot in Russia, has come to Tokyo for a medical examination. He heard from his friend that Japan's medical examinations are high quality and trustworthy. Mr. Antonov wants to know about any possible health problems or risks he might have, so that he can continue to work as a pilot for as long as possible. He is now 38 years old. Mr. Antonov used a travel agency that specializes in medical tourism. He is staying at an international hotel in Kobe, and he visited a few tourist spots in Nara as suggested by his travel agent. During his two-day stay in the hospital, Mr. Antonov will undergo a thorough medical checkup. In the morning of the first day, he finished his chest X-ray and electrocardiogram. In the following dialog, he is going to have a gastroscopy in the afternoon and discusses the lower GI test that will be conducted on the second day.

Patient Information

Name: _____   Nationality: _____

Age: _____   Occupation: _____

Gender: _____   Chief Concerns: _____

1 What is the purpose of Mr. Antonov's visit to Japan?

2 What does Mr. Antonov do?

3 What questions do you think he will ask about his tests?

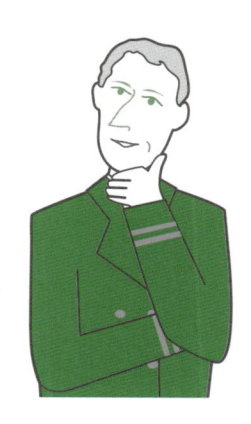

Ⅱ Post-Reading Vocabulary

空欄に入る語をボックスから選び，記号で答えなさい。

1 A ( ) is used to find out if you have any ulcers or cancer in your stomach.

2 Some foreigners visit Japan to receive a thorough, high-quality ( ).

3 A ( ) is an examination of the colon and rectum.

4 An ( ) measures the electrical activity of the heart.

ⓐ medical checkup **ⓑ** electrocardiogram **ⓒ** gastroscopy **ⓓ** lower GI test

---

Ⅲ Pre-Listening Vocabulary

以下の語の定義をボックスから選び，記号で答えなさい。

1 endoscope ( )

2 enema ( )

3 anesthetize ( )

4 laxative ( )

ⓐ a medicine that helps a person to empty their bowels
ⓑ an injection of liquid into the rectum to evacuate the bowels
ⓒ a long thin tube with a small camera
ⓓ to make a person unable to feel pain

Ⅳ Extra Vocabulary (Digestive System)

イラストに対応する語をボックスから選び，記号で答えなさい。

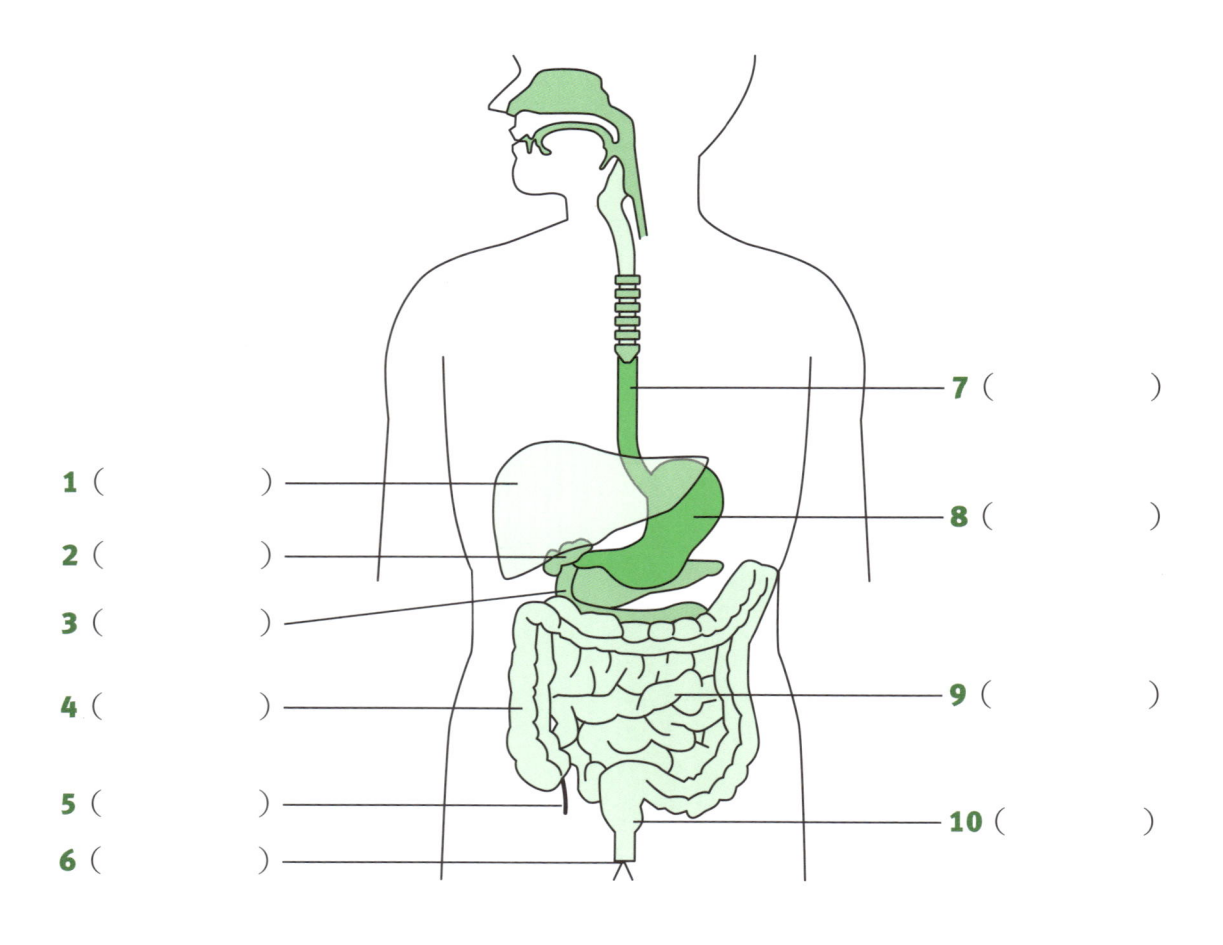

1 (　　　　)

2 (　　　　)

3 (　　　　)

4 (　　　　)

5 (　　　　)

6 (　　　　)

7 (　　　　)

8 (　　　　)

9 (　　　　)

10 (　　　　)

ⓐ esophagus　　ⓑ stomach　　ⓒ duodenum　　ⓓ liver　　ⓔ gallbladder
ⓕ intestine　　ⓖ colon　　ⓗ rectum　　ⓘ anus　　ⓙ appendix

V Listening

看護師と患者さんの会話を聞いて，以下の質問の答えとして最も適切なものを選びなさい。

1 Which part of the body does a gastroscopy examine?
- **ⓐ** stomach
- **ⓑ** intestine
- **ⓒ** mouth
- **ⓓ** rectum

2 How is the tube inserted?
- **ⓐ** through the nose
- **ⓑ** through the mouth
- **ⓒ** through the ear
- **ⓓ** through the anus

3 Which part of the body is anesthetized before inserting the tube?
- **ⓐ** the skin
- **ⓑ** the stomach
- **ⓒ** the duodenum
- **ⓓ** the throat

4 How does Mr. Antonov feel about having an enema?
- **ⓐ** He does not mind it.
- **ⓑ** He wants to avoid it.
- **ⓒ** He doesn't understand what it is.
- **ⓓ** He wants to try it.

5 What is Mr. Antonov supposed to do after 9:00 p.m.?
- **ⓐ** avoid solid foods
- **ⓑ** not eat or drink anything
- **ⓒ** drink plenty of water
- **ⓓ** go to sleep early

Mr. Antonov	I've never had a gastroscopy before. Would you tell me what's going to happen?
Nurse	Sure. The purpose of a gastroscopy is to examine the inside of your stomach. The doctor will insert an endoscope, which is a flexible tube, through your mouth and into your stomach.
Mr. Antonov	Does it hurt?
Nurse	Don't worry, we will anesthetize your throat first, so you won't feel any pain during the procedure. But your throat may be sore for a few days afterward.
Mr. Antonov	I see. Well, let's get it over with!
	[*after the gastroscopy is finished*]
Nurse	Tomorrow you will have your lower GI examination.
Mr. Antonov	Oh. Would you explain it to me?
Nurse	Well, the usual method is a barium enema, which means that white liquid barium is put into your colon using an enema. Then the lining of your colon and rectum can be seen on an X-ray.
Mr. Antonov	Oh, no. I do not like enemas at all.
Nurse	I understand, but we will make sure it is not too uncomfortable. However, if you really want to avoid the enema, you do have the option of doing a colonoscopy instead. It costs quite a bit extra, though.
Mr. Antonov	That sounds better. I'll definitely do that.
Nurse	Please be sure that you do not eat any food between now and your examination tomorrow morning. We'll give you a laxative to take at 9 p.m., and then you can't eat or drink anything after that.
Mr. Antonov	Doing a thorough medical checkup is no fun at all…

Key Expressions

1 The purpose of a gastroscopy is to examine the inside of your stomach.
胃カメラの目的は胃の内部を調べることです。

2 We will anesthetize your throat first, so you won't feel any pain.
最初にのどに麻酔をしますので，痛みはないですよ。

3 We will make sure it is not too uncomfortable.
不快にならないようにしますね。

4 Please be sure that you do not eat any food between now and your examination tomorrow.
今から明日の検査まで何も召し上がらないようにしてください。

5 We'll give you a laxative to take at 9 p.m.
午後9時にはお通じ薬を差し上げます。

Cross-Cultural Topics

人間ドックを説明できますか　A Full Physical Exam Called 'Human Dock'

　日本では，医療保険者に法律で義務付けられた「健康診断（medical examination）」のほかに，身体の健康状態を総合的に診断し，隠れている病気を早期に発見し，生活習慣の改善により病気を予防することを目的とする健康診断「人間ドック」があります。「人間ドック」は，日本生まれの任意型の健康診断で，半日から1日で集中して精密な検査（full physical exam）を行います。

　ちなみに'human dock'という表現は元々の英語にはありません。では，「人間ドック」のドック（dock）はどういう意味でしょうか。英語でドックとは，船を点検・修理したり，荷物の積み下ろしをしたりする場所のことです。1954年（昭和29年），市民が病気を予防するために精密な医療検査を受けられる健康診断が創設され，船が定期的に受ける船全体の精密な点検になぞらえて「人間ドック」と名付けられました。「健康診断」の検査項目は会社・自治体で決まっていますが，「人間ドック」ではより多くの項目について精密な検査を行います。婦人科検診を加えた「レディースドック」など，目的に合わせた検査を行うことも可能です。

　がんや生活習慣病などさまざまな病気の早期発見に貢献する「人間ドック」ですが，健康保険の対象外ですので費用は原則自己負担となります。「健康診断」も「人間ドック」も受けるだけでは意味はありません。健康状態を知り，生活習慣を見直すきっかけとすることで，はじめて病気の予防につながります。「自分の健康は自分で守ること（セルフケア）」が大切なのは世界共通です。

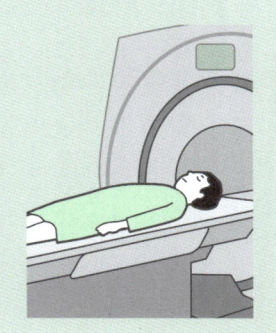

VI Communication Activity
検査の説明をする Instructions for Medical Tests

STEP 1

看護師役と患者さん役に分かれて，以下のモデルダイアローグを練習しましょう。

Example Scenario: Veronika Azarova decided to have a medical checkup in Japan as it is cheaper than in the UK. The nurse is now going to take a blood sample.

Model dialog

Nurse	Ms. Azarova, I am now going to take a blood sample.
Ms. Azarova	OK.
Nurse	First, please put your arm on the armrest.
Ms. Azarova	Which arm? Is my left arm all right? I'm right-handed.
Nurse	No problem. Now make a fist with your thumb inside.
Ms. Azarova	Like this?
Nurse	Yeah, that's right. You will feel a short prick, OK?
Ms. Azarova	All right.
Nurse	All done. Please apply pressure to the bandage for five minutes.
Ms. Azarova	Oh, for such a long time?
Nurse	Well, maybe a bit shorter will be fine if you have no bleeding.

STEP 2

ボックスの中の表現を使って，以下の会話を練習しましょう。

Scenario 1: Steve Brown is a lecturer at a Japanese university, and he needs to have an annual medical checkup. He is now going to have a chest X-ray taken.

Nurse	Mr. Brown, the next test is an X-ray. ① _____
Mr. Brown	Yes, I saw it on the way. Will I have to take off my clothes?
Nurse	Not everything, just your shirt. ② _____
Radiology technician	Mr. Brown, ③ _____
Mr. Brown	All right. I am ready.
Radiology technician	④ _____
Mr. Brown	OK.
Radiology technician	Inhale and hold your breath. Do not move.

ⓐ Come here and stand in front of the X-ray machine.

ⓑ The X-ray technician will help you when you get there.

ⓒ Please take off your shirt and remove all metal items.

ⓓ Do you know how to get to the Radiology Department?

STEP 3

以下の手順に従って，会話の練習をしましょう。

Scenario 2: Brad Clapton is a travel agent, and he has worked in Tokyo for a year. He enjoys going for a drive. Last week, his car was hit from behind. He hit his head hard and was taken to the hospital. The nurse needs to take his vital signs, starting with his blood pressure.

Procedure

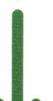

❶ Tell the patient which test is going to be conducted.

❷ Instruct the patient on what to do.

❸ Ask the patient if he/she has any problems or questions.

❹ Tell the patient the test is finished.

Instructions

1 Put your arm here.
2 Make a fist with your thumb inside.
3 Open your hand and relax.
4 Are you allergic to rubbing alcohol?
5 You'll feel a short prick.
6 Do you feel any tingling in your hand or fingers?
7 Press down on the bandage for five minutes.

Other Useful Expressions

1 I'm going to take your blood pressure now.
2 Take a few deep breaths, and try to relax.
3 Roll your sleeve all the way up. A little more, please.
4 I'm just going to wrap this cuff around your arm, OK?
5 You are going to have a CT scan.
6 Please take off all your jewelry and any metallic things.
7 Now please change into this gown.
8 Is everything fine? Do you feel any discomfort?
9 The test will be finished soon. But please do not move yet.
10 Your blood pressure is 130/90 (130 over 90).
11 Now I need to collect a urine sample. First, urinate into the toilet a little, and then fill the cup up to this line.

Departments and Specialists（診療科と専門家医）

1	外科	surgery	surgeon
2	内科	internal medicine	internist
3	整形外科	orthopedics	orthopedist
4	循環器科	cardiology	cardiologist
5	形成外科	plastic surgery	plastic surgeon
6	小児科	pediatrics	pediatrician
7	産科	obstetrics	obstetrician
8	婦人科	gynecology	gynecologist
9	耳鼻咽頭科	otorhinolaryngology / ENT (Ear, Nose and Throat)	otorhinolaryngologist / ENT doctor
10	眼科	ophthalmology	ophthalmologist
11	病理学	pathology	pathologist
12	精神科	psychiatry	psychiatrist
13	神経内科	neurology	neurologist
14	神経外科	neurosurgery	neurosurgeon
15	皮膚科	dermatology	dermatologist
16	放射線科	radiology	radiologist
17	泌尿器科	urology	urologist
18	腫瘍学	oncology	oncologist
19	集中治療室	intensive care unit (ICU)	critical care specialist
20	麻酔科	anesthesiology	anesthesiologist
21	歯科	dentistry	dentist
22	口腔外科	oral surgery	oral surgeon

Women's and Family Health

　このユニットでは，異文化での妊娠，出産や育児という不安やストレスを伴う経験をする外国人女性や家族へのケアについて学びます。グローバル化に伴い，日本各地の市町村で外国語版の母子健康手帳が交付されるようになり，子育て世代の外国人女性や家族への支援の重要性が高まっています。妊娠，出産，育児は，文化によってその方法や習慣が大きく異なるため，異国での生活に加え二重の負担になりがちです。異文化の中で家族が安心して子供を産み育てるために医療者はどのように支援をすればよいのでしょうか。

　ここでは，初めて日本の産婦人科で診察を受ける患者さんと出産を経験する妊婦さん，日本で暮らす外国人夫婦の子供の予防接種の事例を扱います。課題を通して，成育医療のケアに必要なコミュニケーションを学びましょう。

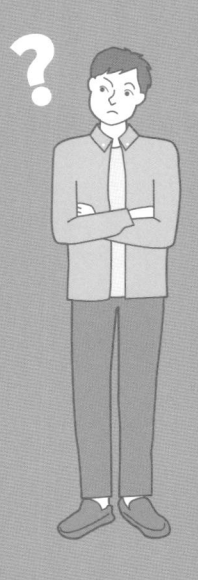

考えてみよう

Q1 多くの外国人女性が日本の婦人科での診療の時に驚くことは何？

Q2 日本では第1子出生時の女性の平均年齢は何歳くらい？アメリカやフランスでは？

Q3 予防接種の記録にもなる「母子手帳」の発祥国はどこで，世界何カ国ぐらいに普及しているの？

Unit 2

Lesson 1

Women's Health

I Reading and Discussion

以下の文章を読んで患者情報を完成させなさい。また，1 ～ 3 の質問に英語で答えなさい。

Kim Suzuki-White is a 33-year-old British lawyer who has worked for a children's charity based in Tokyo since she married her Japanese husband last year. She was diagnosed with endometriosis when she was in her twenties. After her diagnosis she started taking contraceptive pills. Ms. Suzuki-White was on the pill for eight years, but she stopped four months ago because she is trying to get pregnant. Since coming off the pill she has started to experience the symptoms of endometriosis again: painful menstrual periods, lack of energy, and severe lower back pain. During the last three months she has missed several days of work because of the pain. She has come to the clinic today to see what treatments are available to her. This is her first time to come to an OB/GYN clinic in Japan. The gynecologist says she needs an internal exam.

Patient Information

Name: _____

Age: _____

Gender: _____

Marital Status: _____

Nationality: _____

Occupation: _____

Chief Concerns: _____

Medical History: _____

1 Why did Ms. Suzuki-White stop taking contraceptive pills?

2 Why did she come to the clinic?

3 What do you think the nurse should explain to a patient before an internal exam?

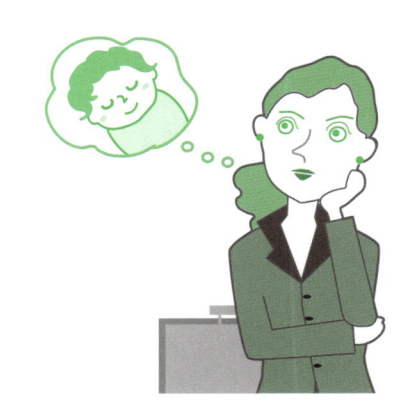

Ⅱ Post-Reading Vocabulary

空欄に入る語をボックスから選び，記号で答えなさい。

1 The doctor will make a (　　　　　) after the examination.

2 Girls usually have their first (　　　　　) around the age of 11 or 12.

3 One of the most common types of birth control is the (　　　　　).

4 The primary symptom of (　　　　　) is severe pelvic pain.

> **ⓐ** diagnosis　　　**ⓑ** endometriosis　　　**ⓒ** contraceptive pill　　　**ⓓ** menstrual period

Ⅲ Pre-Listening Vocabulary

以下の語の定義をボックスから選び，記号で答えなさい。

1 menstrual flow　　　(　　　　　)

2 ultrasound probe　　(　　　　　)

3 internal exam　　　(　　　　　)

4 sanitary pad　　　　(　　　　　)

> **ⓐ** a medical device used to examine the female pelvic organs internally
> **ⓑ** the vaginal bleeding that occurs monthly, lasting for 2-7 days
> **ⓒ** a piece of soft material used by women during menstruation to absorb the uterine flow
> **ⓓ** a physical examination of the female pelvic organs

Ⅳ Extra Vocabulary (Reproductive Organs)

イラストに対応する語をボックスから選び，記号で答えなさい。

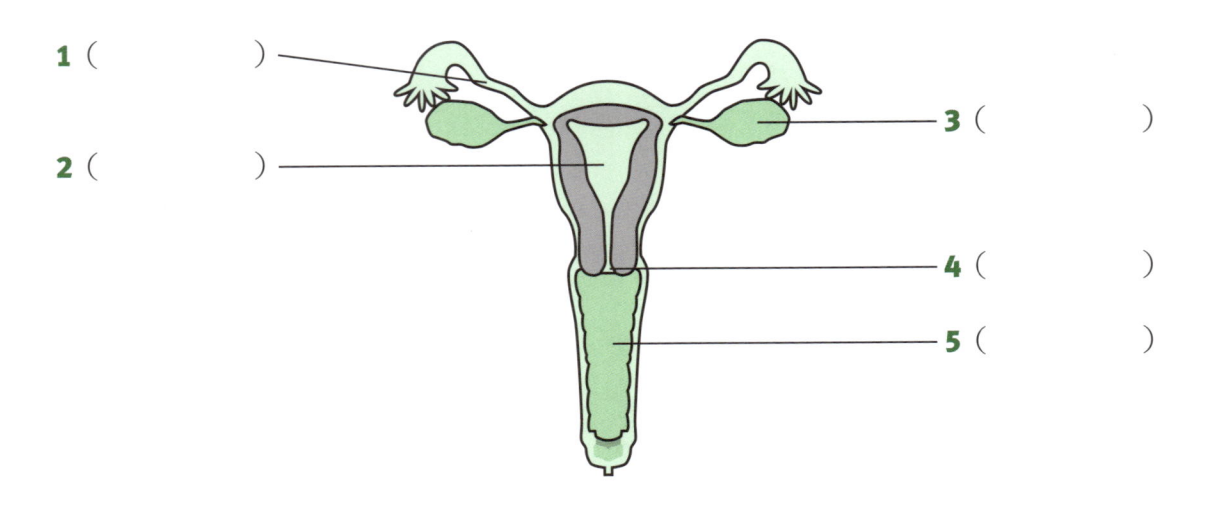

1 (　　　　)

2 (　　　　)

3 (　　　　)

4 (　　　　)

5 (　　　　)

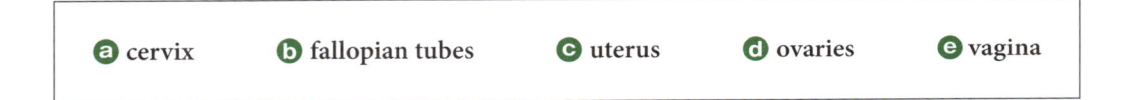

| ⓐ cervix | ⓑ fallopian tubes | ⓒ uterus | ⓓ ovaries | ⓔ vagina |

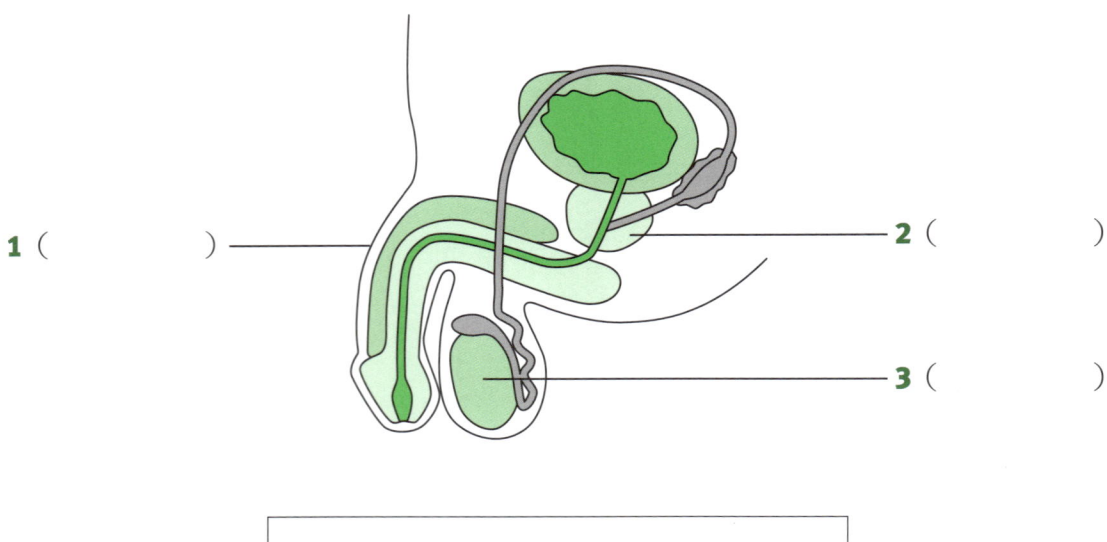

1 (　　　　)

2 (　　　　)

3 (　　　　)

| ⓐ testicle | ⓑ prostate | ⓒ penis |

V Listening

看護師と患者さんの会話を聞いて，以下の質問の答えとして最も適切なものを選びなさい。

1 What question did Ms. Suzuki-White have difficulty completing?

　ⓐ the one about the amount of blood in each period

　ⓑ the one about the date of her last period

　ⓒ the one about the interval between periods

　ⓓ the one about the pain during her period

2 What will NOT be part of her examination with the doctor?

　ⓐ an internal examination

　ⓑ an endoscopy

　ⓒ an ultrasound

　ⓓ questions from the doctor

3 What procedure does Ms. Suzuki-White mention having had before?

　ⓐ a pelvic exam

　ⓑ an external ultrasound

　ⓒ a pregnancy test

　ⓓ a biopsy

4 What kind of doctor does Ms. Suzuki-White request?

　ⓐ an English-speaking doctor

　ⓑ an experienced doctor

　ⓒ a female doctor

　ⓓ a senior doctor

5 Why does Ms. Suzuki-White not want to use the privacy curtain?

　ⓐ She wants to check that the doctor is female.

　ⓑ She wants to see what the doctor is doing.

　ⓒ She thinks having a curtain is a silly idea.

　ⓓ She wants to ask the doctor questions face-to-face.

Nurse	Thank you for filling out the questionnaire. Do you have any questions?
Ms. Suzuki-White	Actually I'm having trouble answering this question about menstrual flow. My period is quite heavy on the second day, but then it is not so bad.
Nurse	Just tick "heavy" and later you can explain it to the doctor.
Ms. Suzuki-White	I see. What kind of examination will I have today?
Nurse	After asking you some questions, the doctor will do a quick pelvic exam. After that he will perform an internal ultrasound scan. Have you had one of those tests before?
Ms. Suzuki-White	I don't think so. I've had an ultrasound on my stomach before, but not internal. What's it like?
Nurse	The doctor will insert an ultrasound probe which uses sound waves to get an image of the uterus. It is painless, but you may find it a little uncomfortable.
Ms. Suzuki-White	Could I be examined by a female doctor?
Nurse	I'm afraid there isn't a woman doctor on duty today. But in the future, you can request a woman doctor if you make an appointment in advance. Is that okay?
Ms. Suzuki-White	Yes, it's okay. What's this curtain?
Nurse	It is a privacy curtain. The doctor will stay behind it so that you can't see him during the exam. Would you like him to use the curtain or not?
Ms. Suzuki-White	No, thank you. I would prefer to see the doctor's face so I can ask him questions if I need to.
Nurse	OK. After the exam, please take a sanitary pad from the basket if you need one.

Key Expressions

1 Thank you for filling out the questionnaire. Do you have any questions?
問診票にご記入くださりありがとうございます。何か質問はありますか。

2 Have you had one of those tests before?
このような検査を以前に受けたことはありますか。

3 It is painless, but you may find it a little uncomfortable.
痛みはありませんが，少し不快感があるかもしれません。

4 I'm afraid there isn't a woman doctor on duty today.
申し訳ありませんが，今日は女性の医師はいません。

5 Would you like him to use the curtain or not?
医師にカーテンを使ってもらいますか。

Cross-Cultural Topics

ウィメンズヘルスと異文化理解　OB/GYN Cultural Considerations

テレビドラマの中の病院の診察室は，海外でも日本でも大きな違いはないように見えます。しかし，外国人患者さんが驚くことが多いのが婦人科の診察室です。日本の病院やクリニックでは患者さんの気持ちを配慮して，診察する医師の顔が見えないよう患者さんと医師の間にカーテンを引くことができる婦人科が多くあります。しかし，このような習慣がない外国人患者さんにとっては医師の姿が見えないカーテン越しの診察は不自然なものであり，不安に思う方もいるかもしれません。カーテンについては，診察の前に必要かどうか確認するとよいでしょう。

患者さんの個人的な希望とは別に，婦人科では宗教上，女性の医師しか受け入れられない場合があることについても理解しておく必要があります。しかし，患者さんの国籍や宗教にかかわらず，検査が必要な場合は，どのような検査を行うのか，検査の方法，その検査が必要な理由を具体的に説明する必要があります。あいまいな説明をしたり，明確な説明がないまま検査に入ったりすると患者さんに大きな不安を与えることになります。検査前に，「これを使いますよ」と使用する検査器具などを患者さんに示し，実際に見てもらっておくことも有効な説明の方法です。

婦人科でも，他の診療科と同様に診察の前には問診の確認をしますが，患者さんが月経サイクルの意味がわからない場合や，外国人患者さんが答えにくい質問事項が含まれている場合がありますので，婦人科では問診におけるナースの役割がいっそう重要であるといえるでしょう。

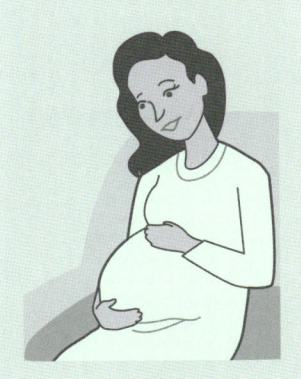

Communication Activity
婦人科の診療の説明をする Explaining a Gynecological Examination

STEP 1

看護師役と患者さん役に分かれて，以下のモデルダイアローグを練習しましょう。

Example Scenario: Jemma Cross is a 17-year-old New Zealand girl. She has come to the clinic because of severe period pain. She has no history of chronic illness.

Model dialog

Nurse Hello. Have you finished filling out the questionnaire?

Ms. Cross I'm having trouble answering these questions about menstruation.

Nurse Just leave them blank and explain it to the doctor.

Ms. Cross What kind of examination will I have today?

Nurse It will be a quick pelvic exam and an internal ultrasound scan. It is painless.

Ms. Cross Thank you.

Nurse There can be a privacy curtain between you and the doctor so you can't see him during the exam. Would you like to use the curtain?

Ms. Cross No, thank you. I don't need the curtain.

STEP 2

ボックスの中の表現を使って，以下の会話を練習しましょう。

Scenario 1: Shelly Lin is a 45-year-old Taiwanese woman. She has come to the clinic because of heavy periods (menorrhagia). She has had mild endometriosis for a few years.

Nurse ① _____

Ms. Lin I'm having trouble answering these questions about menstruation.

Nurse ② _____

Ms. Lin I see. What kind of examination will I have today?

Nurse ③ _____

Ms. Lin Okay.

Nurse ④ _____

Ms. Lin No, thanks. I'll be fine without it.

ⓐ First you will have a quick pelvic exam, and then an internal ultrasound scan.

ⓑ Good morning, were you able to fill out the questionnaire?

ⓒ There is a privacy curtain if you need it.

ⓓ You don't have to answer those now. Just ask the doctor later.

以下の手順に従って，会話の練習をしましょう。

Scenario 2: Kurnia Agustin is a 21-year-old Indonesian student who wears a hijab. Recently her periods have become very irregular. There is no chance that she is pregnant.

Procedure

❶ Greet the patient, and check that all the questions have been answered.

❷ Help the patient with any difficult questions.

❸ Explain what will happen during the examination.

❹ Ask if the patient needs any extra cultural considerations.

Menstrual History Questionnaire

Please check the appropriate boxes.

· When was your first menstrual period?   Age: _____ years old
· When was your menopause?   Age: _____ years old

· How long is your menstrual cycle?
     ☐ 28 days   ☐ 30 days   ☐ _____ days   ☐ Irregular

· On average, how long does your period last?   _____ days

· How heavy is your flow?   ☐ Heavy   ☐ Moderate   ☐ Light

· Do you suffer from menstrual pain?   ☐ Yes   ☐ No

· When was the first day of your last period?
               _____
               Month   Day   Year

Other Useful Expressions

1 If I were you, I would speak to the doctor about that question.
2 You can skip that question for now and ask the doctor later.
3 He will do a quick pelvic exam. After that he will perform an internal ultrasound scan.
4 Do you want to use the privacy curtain?
5 Would you like to be examined by a female doctor?
6 Is there any possibility that you are pregnant?
7 Please sit here and relax.
8 This chair moves automatically and the bottom falls away for the examination.

I Reading and Discussion

以下の文章を読んで患者情報を完成させなさい。また，1〜3の質問に英語で答えなさい。

Dadang and Farah Sudrajat, an Indonesian couple, are the owners of a shop that sells Halal food. They are at Tokyo International Maternity Hospital. Mrs. Sudrajat is 34 years old and this is her third pregnancy. Her first and second pregnancies were uneventful, and she has a 5-year-old daughter and a 3-year-old son. However, Mrs. Sudrajat has had some complications during this pregnancy. She had severe morning sickness in her first trimester, developed gestational diabetes, and suffered from swelling in her ankles, so she is very worried about giving birth. The baby's size is within the normal range. Mrs. Sudrajat's water broke while she was at home. Her husband drove her to the hospital. Like most Muslim men, Mr. Sudrajat did not want to be present at the delivery, so Mrs. Sudrajat went to the delivery room on her own.

Patient Information

Name: _____

Age: _____

Gender: _____

Marital Status: _____

Nationality: _____

Occupation: _____

Chief Concerns: _____

Medical History: _____

1 Why is Mrs. Sudrajat particularly nervous about giving birth?

2 Why did her husband wait outside the delivery room?

3 What extra concern might there be for pregnant women giving birth outside their own country?

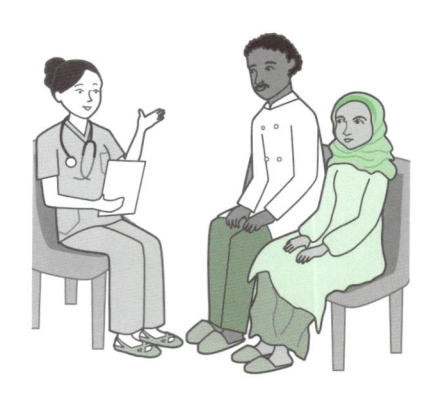

Ⅱ Post-Reading Vocabulary

空欄に入る語をボックスから選び，記号で答えなさい。

1 During pregnancy, many women suffer (　　　　　) of the legs.

2 The main function of a midwife is to provide support and care to women during labor and (　　　　　).

3 In a hospital, medical staff are on standby in case of (　　　　　) during childbirth.

4 If your (　　　　　) breaks, it is necessary to call your midwife or doctor immediately.

ⓐ complications	ⓑ swelling	ⓒ water	ⓓ delivery

Ⅲ Pre-Listening Vocabulary

以下の語の定義をボックスから選び，記号で答えなさい。

1 Apgar score　　　　(　　　　　)

2 contractions　　　　(　　　　　)

3 caesarean section　(　　　　　)

4 epidural　　　　　(　　　　　)

ⓐ an anesthetic procedure used especially in childbirth to produce loss of pain below the waist

ⓑ a surgical incision through the abdominal and uterine walls in order to deliver a baby

ⓒ a measure of the physical condition of an infant at birth

ⓓ strong movements of the uterine muscles that occur during labor

Ⅳ Extra Vocabulary (Stages of Labor)

以下の妊娠段階と対応するイラストを選び，記号で答えなさい。

1 cervix (0 cm)　　　　　　　（　　　　　）
2 cervix dilating　　　　　　（　　　　　）
3 cervix (10 cm) / head turned　（　　　　　）
4 neck flexed　　　　　　　（　　　　　）
5 shoulders emerged　　　　（　　　　　）

ⓐ

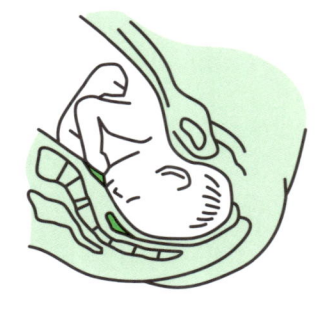

ⓑ

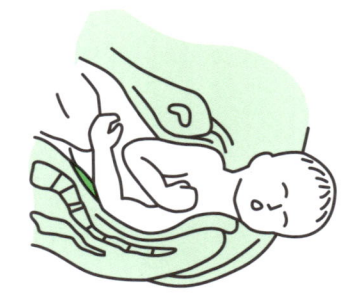

ⓒ

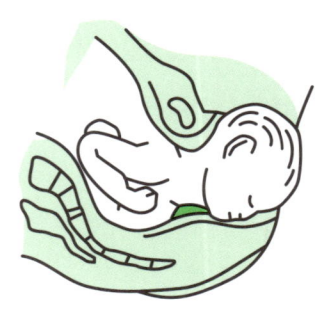

ⓓ

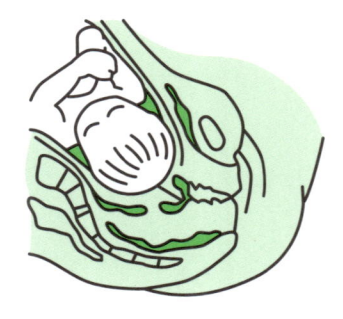

ⓔ

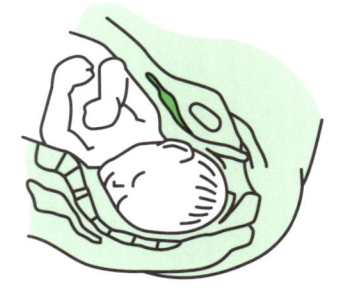

助産師と患者さんの会話を聞いて，以下の質問の答えとして最も適当なものを選びなさい。

1 When did Mrs. Sudrajat's water break?
- ⓐ yesterday
- ⓑ this morning
- ⓒ this afternoon
- ⓓ this evening

2 At the start of the conversation, how many centimeters was Mrs. Sudrajat dilated?
- ⓐ 5 cm
- ⓑ 7 cm
- ⓒ 9 cm
- ⓓ 10 cm

3 What did the midwife do to help Mrs. Sudrajat?
- ⓐ She gave her a massage.
- ⓑ She prepared a hot bath.
- ⓒ She gave her pain medication.
- ⓓ She got some juice for her.

4 Why has Mrs. Sudrajat decided not to use an epidural?
- ⓐ It's too painful.
- ⓑ It's too expensive.
- ⓒ It's not safe.
- ⓓ It's not natural.

5 What did the midwife NOT record as soon as the baby was delivered?
- ⓐ the time of birth
- ⓑ the duration of labor
- ⓒ the baby's weight
- ⓓ the mother's blood loss

Unit 2

Lesson 2

Midwife	When did your water break?
Mrs. Sudrajat	My water broke this afternoon, and I started getting strong contractions early this evening.
Midwife	So that's about four hours ago. Well, you're nine centimeters dilated now. If the pain becomes really bad, let me know and I can give you a back massage.
Mrs. Sudrajat	OK.
Midwife	You've decided not to use an epidural, right?
Mrs. Sudrajat	I would like a natural birth, yes…Oh, here comes another contraction.
Midwife	Let me massage your lower back…. How is that? Is it helping?
Mrs. Sudrajat	Not at all. Oh, no! The pain is becoming really bad. Is it too late for me to ask for a caesarean section?
Midwife	It's definitely too late. Let me just examine you…. OK, the baby's head is crowning now, so it won't be long. I want you to give gentle pushes for now. Then when you feel another contraction coming, I want you to take a deep breath and hold it. Now push hard. Keep pushing…. Keep pushing. Exhale. OK, good work!
Mrs. Sudrajat	I don't think I can do this much longer. It's so painful!
Midwife	You're doing great! Your baby will be delivered on the next contraction. When you feel it, I want you to give me one more really big push…. [*sound of baby crying*] Mrs. Sudrajat, you've got a beautiful baby girl!
Mrs. Sudrajat	That's wonderful!
Midwife	Let me just clean her and check her weight and record the details. Time of birth, 10:07 p.m. Weight, 3,154 grams. Apgar score 8. Blood loss, 300 milliliters. OK, now we'll deliver the placenta and then I'll call your husband to come in.

Key Expressions

1 The baby's head is crowning now, so it won't be long.
赤ちゃんの頭が見えているので，間もなくです。

2 I want you to give gentle pushes for now.
軽くいきんでください。

3 You're doing great! Your baby will be delivered on the next contraction.
とてもいいですよ！　次の収縮で生まれます。

4 I want you to give me one more really big push.
もう一度強くいきんでください。

5 Let me just clean her and check her weight and record the details.
赤ちゃんをきれいにして体重を測り，計測記録をつけます。

Cross-Cultural Topics

女性と家族の健やかな人生を支える助産師　Midwifery around the World

　妊産婦と新生児によりよいケアを提供するという助産師の役割は世界共通といえるでしょう。日本における助産師の歴史は長く，呼び名は時代によって変わってきましたが，常に「女性のそばに寄り添い，女性を励まし，母親と赤ちゃんの安全・安心を守り続けてきた」のが助産師といえます。海外においても，助産師が出産や産前・産後のケアに非常に重要な役割を果たしています。

　例えば，イギリスでは「健康な女性の正常な妊娠および出産においては，助産師が主たるケアの提供者として最もふさわしい」とされており，出産は通常医師ではなく助産師中心に行われます。医療費を国が負担するため，経過が順調であれば出産後1日か2日で退院しなければなりません。日本のように，産後1週間ほど病院において手厚いケアのもと母親が体力を回復し，授乳や沐浴の仕方などを学ぶということはできません。イギリスでは，助産師が家庭を訪問し母子のケアを行うことになります。

　また，同様に出産にかかわる医療費を国が負担するニュージーランドでも大多数の女性が助産師による出産を選択しています。出産を担当した助産師から，週1回ほど産後6週間頃まで継続して訪問を受けることができるシステムになっています。

　しかし，国や地域によっては助産師のケアを受けることができない妊産婦や子供たちがまだ多くいるという現実もあります。助産師の国際的な団体としては，世界中の母親，乳児，家族へのケアの向上を目的として活動する国際助産師連盟（ICM）があり，多くの国から80以上の助産師団体が加入しています。

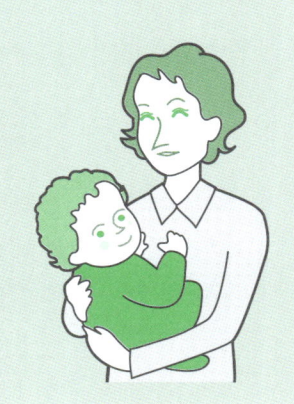

Ⅵ Communication Activity
離乳食指導をする Offering Weaning Advice

助産師役と患者さん役に分かれて，以下のモデルダイアローグを練習しましょう。

Example Scenario: Clare Fowler is Canadian and her daughter Carrie is 6 months old. She has come to the clinic because she is worried about weaning her daughter.

Model dialog

Midwife	Hello, Ms. Fowler. I see you have some questions about your baby's feeding.
Ms. Fowler	Yes. She doesn't seem to like solid food. I'm worried about her weight.
Midwife	I understand. Let's see what we can do. Have you tried giving her some rice porridge puree?
Ms. Fowler	Yes, but she didn't eat much.
Midwife	That's fine. About 2–3 tablespoons of porridge is enough. Even after starting solids, you should breast feed as often as your baby wants it.
Ms. Fowler	Great. How should I cook vegetables for her?
Midwife	Vegetables must be mashed into a soft paste, like mayonnaise.
Ms. Fowler	Do you have any advice about the feeding itself?
Midwife	Be patient. Use gentle and encouraging words while she is eating. If she loses interest while eating, remove other distractions and try to keep her focused.

ボックスの中の表現を使って，以下の会話を練習しましょう。

Scenario 1: John Wilson is from South Africa. His daughter Kylie is 11 months old. Mr. Wilson wants advice about introducing eggs. He is worried about allergies.

Nurse	① _____
Mr. Wilson	I'd like to give Kylie eggs, but I'm worried about allergies.
Nurse	② _____
Mr. Wilson	Okay, thanks. Do you have any advice about other new foods?
Nurse	③ _____
Mr. Wilson	Kelly wants to hold and touch her food. Is that okay?
Nurse	④ _____

> ⓐ Watch her closely for a few days after introducing something new, to check for allergic reactions.
>
> ⓑ Good afternoon. What brings you to the clinic today?
>
> ⓒ No problem at all. It's important to let your child touch the food before eating.
>
> ⓓ You should be able to give her boiled egg yolk now, but consult your doctor if you are worried.

STEP 3

以下の手順に従って，会話の練習をしましょう。

Scenario 2: Tran Mai is Vietnamese. Her 9-month-old son Bao's teeth are coming through. Her mother-in-law suggested giving him some meat, but Mrs. Mai is worried about him choking.

Procedure

❶ Greet the parent/guardian and ask how you can help.

❷ Give advice on what kind of food to give.

❸ Give advice on how often and how much food to give.

❹ Explain how to encourage the infant to eat.

Stages of Feeding

When	What	How
5-6 months Puree 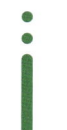	· Rice porridge puree · Soft vegetable paste · Mashed tofu or whitefish	· Breast feed 'on demand' (as often as your baby wants it). · Start offering two-three tablespoons of food about three times per day. · Increase the amount offered gradually.
6-8 months Soft enough to be crushed with the tongue	· Rice porridge or bread porridge · Pureed fruits (bananas, apple) and vegetables (carrots, peas, potatoes) · Pea-sized pieces of meat or fish · Boiled egg yolk / tofu · Yogurt	· Increase the amount and variety of baby foods according to your baby's stool and appetite. · Try to feed your baby at the same times every day to create a daily routine. · Enjoy eating with the whole family.
9-11 months Soft enough to be gummed	· Rice porridge or soft rice · Mashed fruits and vegetables · Boiled egg yolk / tofu · Tiny pieces of meat or fish · Whole eggs · Small amounts of any pasteurized cheese · Heated cow's milk	· Feed your baby three-four times a day, preferably at the same times. · It's common for babies to eat about a ½ cup of food at each meal. · Allow additional snacks if your baby wants them. · Let your baby hold or touch what s/he is eating. · Don't worry about messes—let your child enjoy learning about food.

Additional precautions:
· Don't give your child honey before 12 months of age.
· Never give peanuts as there is a choking risk.

Other Useful Expressions

1 Mash or finely chop food to help him feed himself.

2 It you cut it into tiny pieces, your baby shouldn't choke. Enjoy dinner together!

3 Meats are a good source of iron, particularly for breastfed babies.

4 It's okay to breastfeed if your baby doesn't like solid food while teething.

Unit 2 · Lesson 3

Children's Health

I Reading and Discussion

以下の文章を読んで患者情報を完成させなさい。また，1〜3の質問に英語で答えなさい。

Jim Stanford is a 38-year-old American engineer living in Japan. He and his Korean wife have one son who is 4 months old. Mr. Stanford and his wife share child care responsibilities, so today he has brought his son to the clinic for his vaccinations. The child, Brandon, has had no illnesses since birth. He is feeding well and has had normal weight gain. Mr. Stanford has been given an English version of the vaccine screening questionnaire because he cannot read Japanese. Today, Brandon will be getting his second dose of the DPT-IPV and the third dose of both the Hib and PCV vaccinations. There is no need for payment for any of the doses or booster shots of the routine vaccinations series when carried out within the time schedule. The cost is covered by the government. Mr. Stanford has received a notice of those vaccinations from the local municipal health center, so he brought that as well as his Mother and Child Health Handbook.

Patient Information

Name: _____ Occupation: _____

Age: _____ Chief Concerns: _____

Gender: _____ Medical History: _____

Nationality: _____

1 How many vaccinations in total will Brandon have this visit?

2 What did Mr. Stanford bring to the clinic?

3 What do you think the nurse needs to explain to the patient's guardian before the injection?

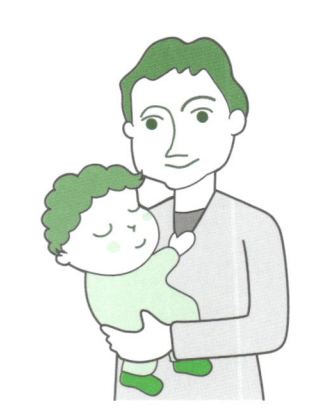

Ⅱ Post-Reading Vocabulary

空欄に入る語をボックスから選び，記号で答えなさい。

1 It is very important to ensure that a child's (　　　　) are up to date.

2 Many immunizations require a (　　　　) when the child is older.

3 The Hib vaccine is delivered in three (　　　　).

4 The (　　　　) protects children from four infectious diseases.

ⓐ vaccinations	ⓑ doses	ⓒ booster shot	ⓓ DPT-IPV

Ⅲ Pre-Listening Vocabulary

以下の語の定義をボックスから選び，記号で答えなさい。

1 side effect　　　　(　　　　)

2 injection　　　　(　　　　)

3 allergic reaction　(　　　　)

4 BCG　　　　　　(　　　　)

ⓐ bacillus Calmette-Guérin, a vaccine against tuberculosis

ⓑ a secondary, undesirable effect of a drug or medical treatment

ⓒ an overreaction of the body's immune system to a food or substance

ⓓ the act of putting a drug into the body by means of a syringe

Ⅳ Extra Vocabulary (Vaccination)

ボックスにある語を使って，表を完成させなさい。

Type of Vaccination	Disease Prevented
Hib（Haemophilus influenzae type b）vaccine	Hib 感染症（細菌性髄膜炎）
PCV（Pneumococcal conjugate vaccine）	肺炎球菌感染症（肺炎，髄膜炎，中耳炎など）
BCG	結核
DPT-IPV （①＿＿＿＿＿, ②＿＿＿＿＿, ③＿＿＿＿＿, ④＿＿＿＿＿ vaccine）	①ジフテリア ②百日せき ③破傷風 ④不活化ポリオ
MR（⑤＿＿＿＿＿ & ⑥＿＿＿＿＿）	⑤麻しん ⑥風しん
⑦＿＿＿＿＿＿	⑦日本脳炎
⑧＿＿＿＿＿＿	⑧水痘（水ぼうそう）

a measles	**b** tetanus	**c** diphtheria	**d** Japanese encephalitis
e chickenpox	**f** inactivated polio	**g** rubella (German measles)	
h pertussis (whooping cough)			

看護師と患者さんの会話を聞いて，以下の質問の答えとして最も適当なものを選びなさい。

1 What vaccination will Brandon NOT get today?

  a PCV

  b DTP-IPV

  c Hib

  d MR

2 What does the nurse NOT need from Mr. Stanford now?

  a a notice from the municipal health center

  b the Mother and Child Health Handbook

  c payment

  d the screening questionnaire

3 Which is a possible side effect of today's vaccinations?

  a swelling around the injection site

  b rapid weight loss

  c problems with vision

  d dizziness

4 Why does the nurse want Brandon to stay in the clinic after the injection?

  a to give her time to translate the questionnaire

  b to make sure his credit card payment goes through

  c to perform a second examination

  d to ensure there are no severe side effects

5 What is the reason for Mr. Stanford's reluctance to give his son the BCG vaccination?

  a It is expensive.

  b There are possible side effects.

  c The procedure will take too long.

  d It is not required in his home country.

▶ Dialog

Nurse	So, you are here for the second dose of the DPT-IPV and the third dose of the Hib and the PCV vaccine today, right?
Mr. Stanford	Yes, here is Brandon's Mother and Child Handbook. And here is the vaccination notice from the local municipal health center.
Nurse	All right. Routine vaccinations are all free of charge. I need you to fill out this vaccine screening questionnaire.
Mr. Stanford	OK. [*after filling out the form*] Here you are.
Nurse	Let's see…. Brandon had his second dose of the Hib and PCV vaccination one month ago, right?
Mr. Stanford	Yes, that's right.
Nurse	This sheet explains the most common side effects. There might be some redness or swelling around the injection site, loss of appetite, and perhaps difficulty sleeping.
Mr. Stanford	Can we leave right after the injection?
Nurse	We will ask you to stay in the clinic for about 30 minutes after the injection just to make sure there is no severe allergic reaction. It's very rare, but just to be safe.
Mr. Stanford	OK. Actually I had another question, about the BCG. In the US it is not required. Does Brandon really need to have it?
Nurse	You should ask the doctor about that. She will be ready in a minute, so please have a seat until your name is called…OK, the doctor will see you now.

Key Expressions

1 I need you to fill out this vaccine screening questionnaire.
問診票に記入してもらう必要があります。

2 This sheet explains the most common side effects.
この紙には一般的な（予防接種の）副作用の説明が書かれています。

3 There might be some redness or swelling around the injection site.
接種部分が赤くなったり腫れたりすることがあるかもしれません。

4 We will ask you to stay in the clinic for about 30 minutes after the injection just to make sure there is no severe allergic reaction.
重いアレルギー反応が出ないか様子をみるために，接種後 30 分はクリニックにいてください。

5 It's very rare, but just to be safe.
めったにはないことですが，念のためです。

6 You should ask the doctor about that.
それについては医師にたずねてください。

Cross-Cultural Topics

相手の立場に立ったコミュニケーション
Cultural Competence in Clinical Communication

　子供の病に向き合い，異文化での慣れない病院生活の中で大きなストレスを抱えている家族に，医療上の清潔の概念を理解してもらい，さらに行動に移してもらうことはなかなか難しいことです。

　子供の病気によっては，入院中に子供に付き添う家族が菌を持ち込まないように気をつけてもらう必要があります。しかし，文化によっては，右手は神聖な手であるため，その手を消毒しなければならないことの意味を理解しにくい場合もあります。また，日本人と同様に部屋の中では靴を履かない習慣をもつ国の人々は病室で素足や靴下で過ごし，そのまま子供に添い寝をする場合などがあります。そのような場合，十分なコミュニケーションを取りながら，相手の文化や習慣を尊重しつつ，同時に清潔を保ってもらえる方法を一緒に見つけていくことが大切だと言えます。

　医療上，重大な場面で家族とのコミュニケーションに困難を感じることがあれば，言葉の支援を行う支援員（医療通訳など）の力を借り，子供にとって安全で最善のケアを提供することが必要です。言葉の上でのコミュニケーションに支障がないと思えるような場合も，実は遠慮から問題や悩みを訴えられずにいる可能性もありますので，細やかなコミュニケーションを図るよう心がけたいものです。外国からの患者さん向けの医療通訳やサポートのボランティアの活用についても，必要に応じて情報を提供するなど，多方面からの支援を可能にすることも家族にとって大きな助けとなるでしょう。

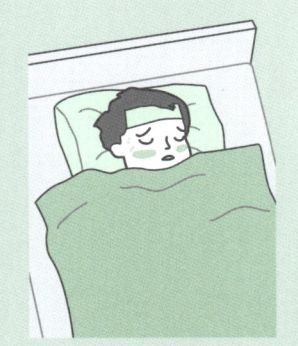

VI Communication Activity
予防接種の説明をする Explaining Vaccinations

STEP 1

看護師役と患者さん役に分かれて，以下のモデルダイアローグを練習しましょう。

Example Scenario: Tessa Next has brought her 5-month-old son Matthew to the clinic to get the third dose of the DPT-IPV vaccination.

Model dialog

Nurse Hello. I need your Mother and Child Health Handbook to record the vaccination.

Ms. Next Here it is.

Nurse Thanks. Please fill out this vaccine screening questionnaire and sign it at the bottom. Do you have any questions?

Ms. Next Is it okay to give my son a bath tonight?

Nurse Bathing is fine, but you shouldn't rub the injection site.

Ms. Next I see.

Nurse Okay, I just need to take the baby's temperature. Could you hold this thermometer under the baby's arm please? How has your child been recently?

Ms. Next He's been pretty good [*takes the baby's temperature*]. Here you are.

Nurse Thank you. The doctor will be ready in a minute, so please have a seat until your name is called.

STEP 2

ボックスの中の表現を使って，以下の会話を練習しましょう。

Scenario 1: Sabine Gröne has brought her 2-month-old son Lucas to the clinic to get the first dose of the Hib vaccination. She wants to know if it is okay to leave the clinic immediately after the vaccination, as she has another appointment.

Nurse ① _____

Ms. Gröne Yes, here it is. Can I leave here immediately after the vaccination?

Nurse ② _____

Ms. Gröne I see.

Nurse ③ _____

Ms. Gröne He has been great. Here you are.

Nurse ④ _____

ⓐ Please wait in the waiting area until your name is called.

ⓑ I just need to take the baby's temperature. [*Give her the thermometer*] How has your son been lately?

ⓒ Good afternoon, do you have the Mother and Child Health Handbook?

ⓓ No, you shouldn't. You need to stay here for 30 minutes or ensure that you can contact the clinic.

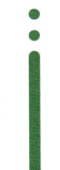

以下の手順に従って，会話の練習をしましょう。

Senario 2: Jeremy Cameron has brought his 6-year-old daughter Samantha to the clinic to get the second dose of the MR vaccine. She is on a soccer team, so he wants to know if she can go to practice today.

Procedure

1. Greet the parent/guardian, ask for the Mother and Child Health Handbook, and give him/her the vaccine screening questionnaire.
2. Explain what they should NOT to do after the injection.
3. Take the child's temperature and check the infant's general condition.
4. Ask them to wait for their names to be called.

Unit 2

Lesson 3

Points to Confirm Before a Child's Vaccination

1 Check that child's temperature is below 37.5°C.

2 Explain the benefits and the risks of the vaccination.

3 Make sure that the guardian agrees to get the child vaccinated.

4 Collect the questionnaire and answer any questions.

5 Collect the Mother and Child Health Handbook.

What to Expect After Vaccinations

1 Wait in the clinic for at least 30 minutes.

There is a very small chance of a severe reaction to the vaccination immediately afterwards, so you need to stay in the clinic for 30 minutes after the injection, or to ensure that you can contact the clinic.

2 Avoid any heavy physical exercise.

Other possible side effects of vaccinations include redness or swelling around the injection site, loss of appetite, or fever. We recommend that you avoid intense activities on the day of vaccination and don't irritate the injection site.

3 Do not give any medicine containing aspirin.

If your child does develop a fever, do NOT give him/her Bufferin or any medicine containing aspirin. Keep the child cool and provide enough to drink. If the fever does not go down, or you have any other concerns, please contact the clinic as soon as possible.

Doctors（医師）

1	医師	physician
2	内科医	internist, physician
3	外科医	surgeon
4	研修医	resident
5	担当医	attending physician, doctor in charge
6	歯科医師	dentist

Nurses（看護師）

1	看護師	registered nurse （RN）
2	准看護師	associate nurse
3	看護助手	nursing assistant, nurse's aide
4	助産師	midwife
5	保健師	public health nurse
6	訪問看護師	visiting nurse
7	養護教諭	school nurse
8	専門看護師	clinical nurse specialist (CNS)
9	認定看護師	certified nurse

Allied Health Professionals（コメディカル）

1	薬剤師	pharmacist
2	管理栄養士	registered dietitian
3	臨床検査技師	clinical laboratory technician
4	放射線技師	X-ray technician
5	理学療法士	physical therapist/physiotherapist
6	作業療法士	occupational therapist
7	言語聴覚士	speech-language-hearing therapist
8	視能訓練士	eye specialist/orthoptist
9	歯科衛生技師	dental hygienist
10	臨床心理士	clinical psychotherapist
11	医療ソーシャルワーカー	medical social worker
12	精神保健福祉士	psychiatric social worker
13	救急救命士	paramedic, emergency medical technician (EMT)
14	医療通訳	medical interpreter
15	牧師（病院付きの）	chaplain

Chronic Illness

　このユニットでは，異文化において長期間の治療が必要な慢性病に向き合う患者さんとその家族へのケアについて学びます。慢性疾患のうち，糖尿病，高血圧，がん，心疾患，脳血管疾患などの生活習慣病（lifestyle-related disease）は，日本でも深刻な健康問題であり，徐々に進行していく病に日々向き合う患者さんとその家族は大きな不安を抱えて日々の治療に臨んでいます。では，異文化の中で，この不安に向き合いながら治療を受ける外国人患者さんとその家族に対して，医療従事者はどのように接すればよいのでしょうか。

　ここでは，特に狭心症，腎不全，認知症を抱える患者さんの事例を扱います。課題を通して，慢性病をかかえる患者さんのQOLを向上させるにはどうすればよいか学びましょう。

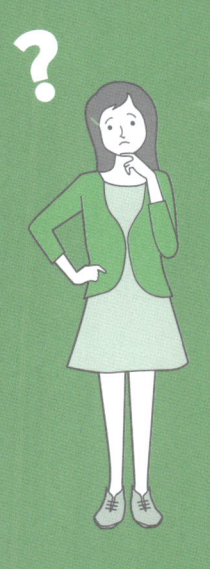

考えてみよう

Q1 慢性病の死因の８割を占める
４つの慢性疾患は何？

Q2 糖尿病の死亡率，
多いのは先進国，発展途上国？

Q3 認知症の危険因子となる生活習慣とは？

Lifestyle-Related Disease

I Reading and Discussion

以下の文章を読んで患者情報を完成させなさい。また，1～3の質問に英語で答えなさい。

One morning, Min Wang, a Chinese woman aged 45, visits Dr. Okano's clinic, which specializes in chronic disease, to consult with him about her recent health problems. She has been experiencing severe palpitations and also having trouble breathing. The day before yesterday, she had a terrible pain in her chest. Mrs. Wang works at a Chinese restaurant with her husband, who is the chef and owner. She used to help during the busy lunchtime rush, but these days she finds it difficult to work for even a few hours. She has been obese since the birth of her second baby in her early thirties, and she was diagnosed with angina pectoris three years ago. Having waited for half an hour after filling out the medical questionnaire, Mrs. Wang is visibly irritated and asks a nurse why she has to wait so long.

Patient Information

Name: _____

Age: _____

Gender: _____

Marital Status: _____

Nationality: _____

Occupation: _____

Chief Concerns: _____

Recent Health Problems: _____

Medical History: _____

1 Summarize the patient's current symptoms.

2 Why is the patient irritated?

3 How do you think the nurse should respond to this patient?

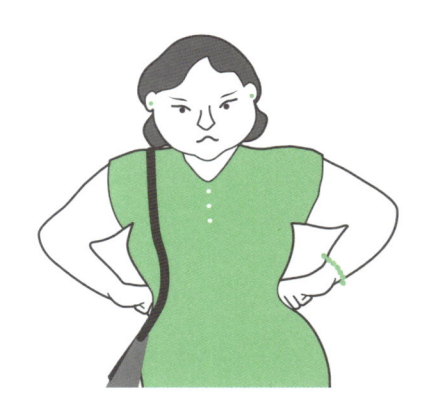

Ⅱ Post-Reading Vocabulary

空欄に入る語をボックスから選び，記号で答えなさい。

1 The patient complained of severe (　　　　　　), which are often a warning of heart disease.

2 More than one-third of Americans are clinically defined as (　　　　　　).

3 (　　　　　　) is a serious type of chest pain caused by not having enough blood flowing to the heart.

4 Asthma is a common (　　　　　　) treated by doctors.

ⓐ angina pectoris　　　**ⓑ** palpitations　　　**ⓒ** chronic disease　　　**ⓓ** obese

---

Ⅲ Pre-Listening Vocabulary

以下の語の定義をボックスから選び，記号で答えなさい。

1 lifestyle-related disease　(　　　　　)

2 consulting room　　　　　(　　　　　)

3 bypass surgery　　　　　 (　　　　　)

4 diet　　　　　　　　　　(　　　　　)

ⓐ the kind of food that a person, animal, or community usually eats

ⓑ the place where a doctor or other therapeutic practitioner examines patients

ⓒ an operation that reroutes the blood flow around blockages in the arteries

ⓓ a disease associated with the way a person lives, such as heart disease, stroke, obesity, type 2 diabetes, etc.

Ⅳ Extra Vocabulary (Circulatory System)

イラストに対応する語をボックスから選び，記号で答えなさい。

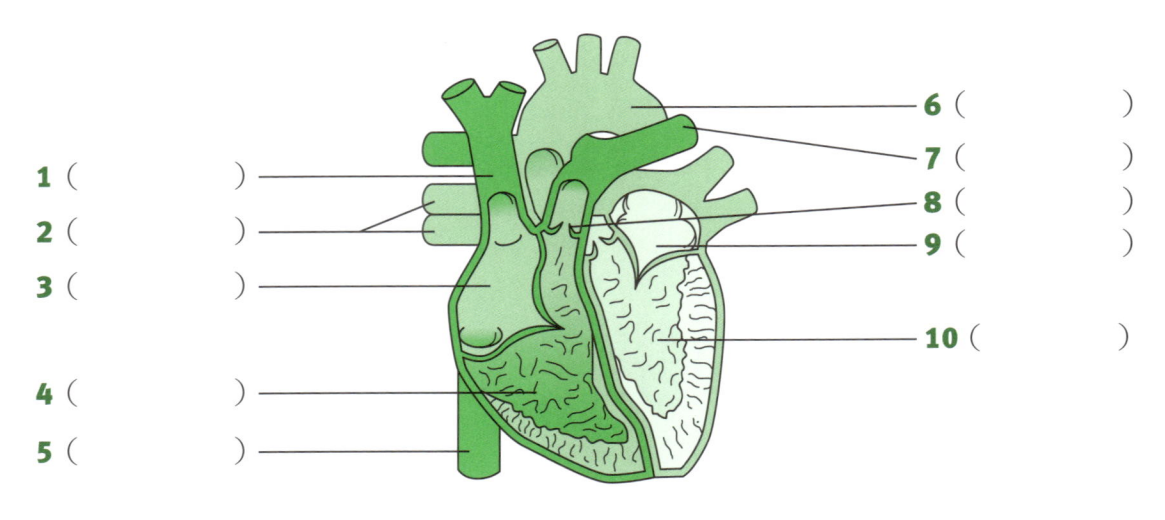

1 (　　　　)
2 (　　　　)
3 (　　　　)
4 (　　　　)
5 (　　　　)

6 (　　　　)
7 (　　　　)
8 (　　　　)
9 (　　　　)
10 (　　　　)

ⓐ superior vena cava	ⓑ inferior vena cava	ⓒ left atrium	ⓓ right atrium
ⓔ left ventricle	ⓕ right ventricle	ⓖ pulmonary veins	
ⓗ pulmonary arteries	ⓘ aorta	ⓙ valve	

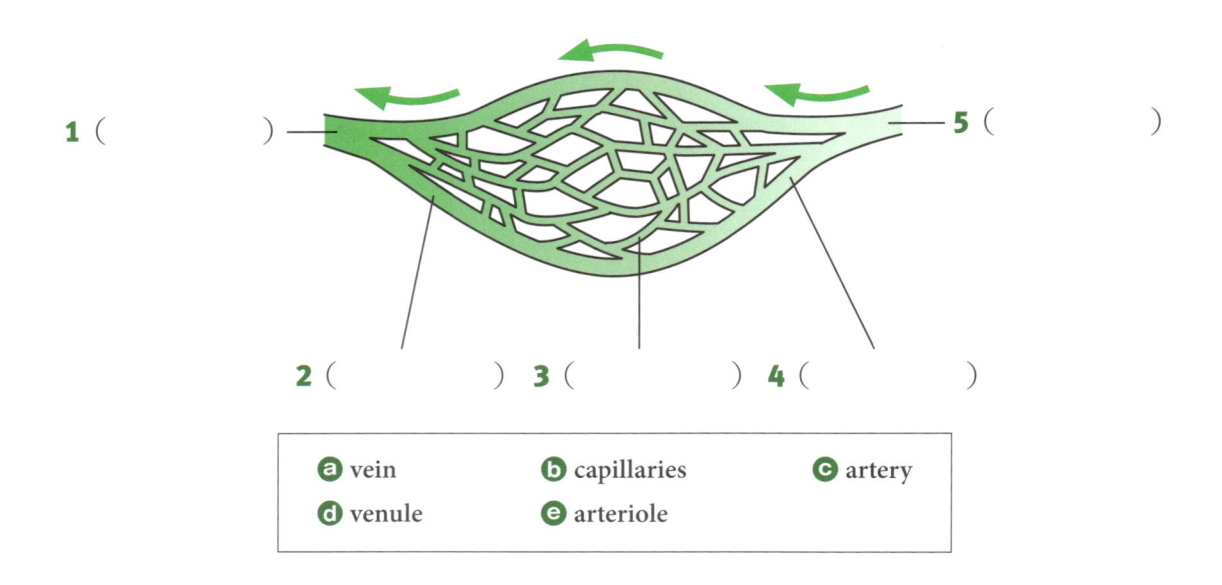

1 (　　　　)
5 (　　　　)

2 (　　　　)　3 (　　　　)　4 (　　　　)

ⓐ vein	ⓑ capillaries	ⓒ artery
ⓓ venule	ⓔ arteriole	

V | Listening

看護師と患者さんの会話を聞いて，以下の質問の答えとして最も適当なものを選びなさい。

1 Why did the patient complain?
- ⓐ The nurse asked her too many questions.
- ⓑ The nurse was rude to foreign patients.
- ⓒ The waiting room was too crowded.
- ⓓ It took a long time for her to see a doctor.

2 Why is the clinic especially busy today?
- ⓐ It is influenza season.
- ⓑ It is the beginning of the week.
- ⓒ It is the end of the month.
- ⓓ They do not have enough doctors on duty.

3 Why were some patients leaving earlier even though they had arrived later?
- ⓐ They made an appointment in advance.
- ⓑ Those who were in a hurry cancelled their examination.
- ⓒ Some patients had different needs.
- ⓓ Important patients were immediately attended to.

4 How long would Mrs. Wang have to stay in the hospital if she had bypass surgery?
- ⓐ about 10 days
- ⓑ about 14 days
- ⓒ about 18 days
- ⓓ about 21 days

5 Which advice did the nurse NOT mention regarding the patient's lifestyle?
- ⓐ Avoid stressful situations.
- ⓑ Do regular exercise.
- ⓒ Avoid unhealthy food.
- ⓓ Stop smoking.

Unit 3

Lesson 1

Dialog

Mrs. Wang   Nurse, I've been waiting here for such a long time. I really can't wait any longer.

Nurse   We are very sorry to have kept you waiting. It's the beginning of the week, so we have more patients than usual.

Mrs. Wang   I've seen some people who came later than me leave earlier. Why is that?

Nurse   Well, we sometimes change the order depending on each patient's needs. For example, some patients just come to pick up a prescription for their regular medication.

Mrs. Wang   Do they? How many more people are before me?

Nurse   Let me see here…. Mrs. Wang, you have just two more patients ahead of you.

Mrs. Wang   All right. That's not so bad.

Nurse   Please wait for a while in front of Consulting Room 3 at the end of the hall.

[*After the examination.*]

Nurse   Mrs. Wang, as Dr. Okano told you, you may need bypass surgery if your symptoms do not improve in the next few months.

Mrs. Wang   Yes, I know. How long will I have to stay in the hospital if I have surgery?

Nurse   Probably about two weeks, but we still can avoid that if you change your lifestyle.

Mrs. Wang   Is that so? What kind of changes?

Nurse   Well, exercising daily and eating a healthy diet are the two most important things.

Mrs. Wang   I've certainly heard that before. What else?

Nurse   Also, you should try to avoid too much stress. Please read this brochure about how to manage lifestyle-related diseases.

Key Expressions

1 We are very sorry to have kept you waiting.
お待たせしてしまい，申し訳ありません。

2 We sometimes change the order depending on each patient's needs.
それぞれの患者さんの必要性に応じて，順番が変わることもあります。

3 You have just two more patients ahead of you.
もうあと 2 人の患者さんの次になります。

4 Please wait for a while in front of Consulting Room 3 at the end of the hall.
廊下の突き当たりの診察室 3 の前でしばらくお待ちください。

5 Exercising daily and eating a healthy diet are the two most important things.
毎日の運動と健康的な食事が最も重要な 2 つの要素です。

Unit 3

Lesson 1

Cross-Cultural Topics

行列大国ニッポン "I've been waiting for a long time!"

　海外の人気観光地で行列に並んでいて横入りされたという経験はありませんか。ランチに 1 時間，ラーメン一杯に 2 時間，アトラクションに乗るために 3，4 時間と，横入りも喧嘩も起こらず，整然と並ぶ日本人の姿は外国人には奇異に映るかもしれません。「行列大国日本」では病院も例外ではありません。「3 時間待って 3 分診療」と揶揄されてきた都市部の大病院でも患者さんはひたすら我慢強く待つことに慣れています。国民皆保険制度が整い，全員を公平に診察する日本の医療では first-come-first-served（先着順）の原則で診療が行われているために，予約があっても診察が長引けば後の患者さんはその分だけ待つことになります。ホームドクター（家庭医，GP）制度が整っている欧米では状況は異なります。特にイギリスでは登録された家庭医が担う役割が大きく，患者さんが地域の拠点病院や大学病院に行く機会は限られているのです。

　受診するためにどれくらい待つことができるかという「医療待ち時間」は，母国での経験によっても異なります。もし待っている外国人患者さんからクレームがきたら，状況を説明して理解を得ることが重要です。医療従事者は患者さんの症状を見極めながら誠意をもって対応することが求められます。

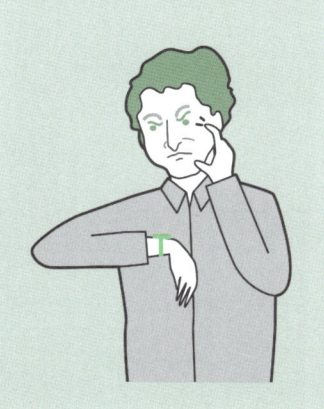

VI Communication Activity
院内の案内をする（フロアマップ参照）Giving Directions

STEP 1

看護師役と患者さん役に分かれて，以下のモデルダイアローグを練習しましょう。

Example Scenario: Michael Thomas, 60 years of age, is coughing persistently. He needs to have an X-ray, but cannot find the way to the Radiology Department. The nurse finds Mr. Thompson wandering around near the entrance.

Model dialog

Nurse [*at the entrance*] Hello, are you looking for something?

Mr. Thomas Yes, I need to have my chest X-rayed in the Radiology Department. I can't find it.

Nurse All right. Please turn left at the first corner there, and go down the hall.

Mr. Thomas OK. And then?

Nurse Radiology is at the end of the hall on your left across from Cardiology.

Mr. Thomas Much appreciated.

Nurse No problem. You seem to have a terrible cough, though. Here is a mask. Please take care of yourself.

STEP 2

ボックスの中の表現を使って，以下の会話を練習しましょう。

Scenario 1: Jane Brown, 50 years old, who has been troubled by dermatitis for the past few weeks, has come to this hospital for the first time. She is looking for the Dermatology Department, but she can't find it on the map shown at the reception desk.

Nurse ① _____

Mrs. Brown Oh, thank you. That's very kind of you. I was told to go to Dermatology.

Nurse ② _____

Mrs. Brown I see. And then?

Nurse ③ _____

Mrs. Brown That sounds easy enough. Thank you so much.

Nurse ④ _____

ⓐ Get off the elevator and go to the right. Turn left at the first corner. Dermatology will be on your left.

ⓑ Excuse me, but do you need any help finding your way?

ⓒ You can't miss it. Please ask any of our staff if you need further help.

ⓓ OK. First, take the elevator to the second floor.

以下の手順に従って，会話の練習をしましょう。

Scenario 2: Kate McDowell, age 24, is suffering from insomnia. She wants to consult with a psychiatrist. Now, she is having trouble getting to the Mental Health Clinic.

Procedure

❶ Greet and ask patient's destination.

❷ Give instructions on how to get there.

❸ Give further explanation, if needed.

❹ Send the patient off with considerate comments.

You are at the Entrance.

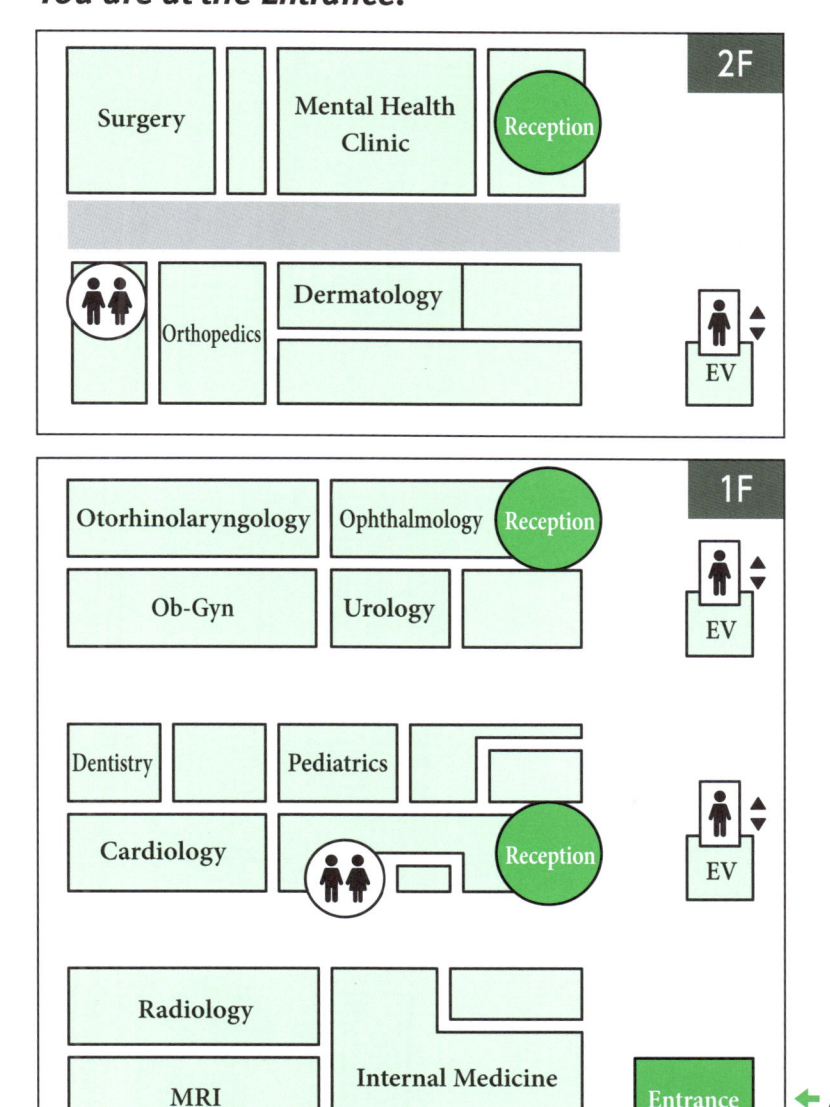

Unit 3

Lesson 2

Dietary Restrictions

I Reading and Discussion

以下の文章を読んで患者情報を完成させなさい。また，1～3 の質問に英語で答えなさい。

Elizabeth Spencer, a British woman who is a 55-year-old widow, has come to the hospital for dialysis. She has been undergoing this treatment since she was diagnosed with kidney failure two years ago. She has dialysis three times a week. Because of her non-adherence to the doctor's dietary restrictions, she has recently been experiencing some confusion. The doctor in charge recommends more frequent dialysis treatments. However, Mrs. Spencer says that that would be difficult. She does not have time because she often has to take care of her granddaughter. The doctor says that if her condition does not improve, she will have to receive a kidney transplant. The nurse gives her advice about dietary changes she can make in order to improve her condition.

Patient Information

Name: _____

Age: _____

Gender: _____

Nationality: _____

Chief Concerns: _____

Medical History: _____

1 Why did this patient come to the hospital?

2 How does the patient's worsening condition affect her QOL?

3 What dietary advice do you think the nurse will offer?

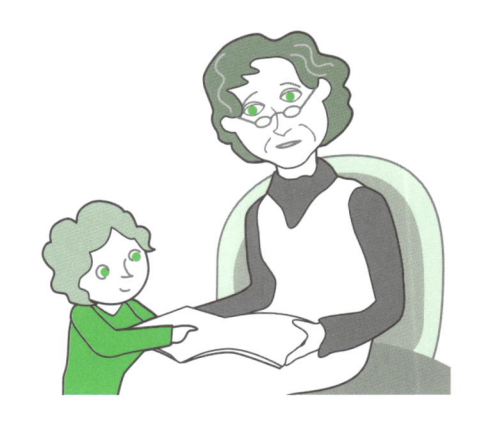

Ⅱ Post-Reading Vocabulary

空欄に入る語をボックスから選び，記号で答えなさい。

1 Her condition requires weekly (　　　　　　) to remove impurities from the blood.

2 His family has been helping him follow strict (　　　　　　) since the onset of his disease.

3 (　　　　　　) is one of the leading causes of death among diabetics.

4 Patients' (　　　　　　) to doctors' advice often worsens their condition.

> **ⓐ** dietary restrictions　　**ⓑ** dialysis　　**ⓒ** kidney failure　　**ⓓ** non-adherence

Ⅲ Pre-Listening Vocabulary

以下の語の定義をボックスから選び，記号で答えなさい。

1 underweight　　　　(　　　　　　)

2 confusion　　　　　(　　　　　　)

3 low-sodium diet　　(　　　　　　)

4 shortness of breath　(　　　　　　)

> **ⓐ** uncertainty about what is happening
> **ⓑ** eating only foods with little or no salt
> **ⓒ** feeling like you can't get enough air
> **ⓓ** below a normal or desirable weight

イラストに対応する語をボックスから選び，記号で答えなさい。

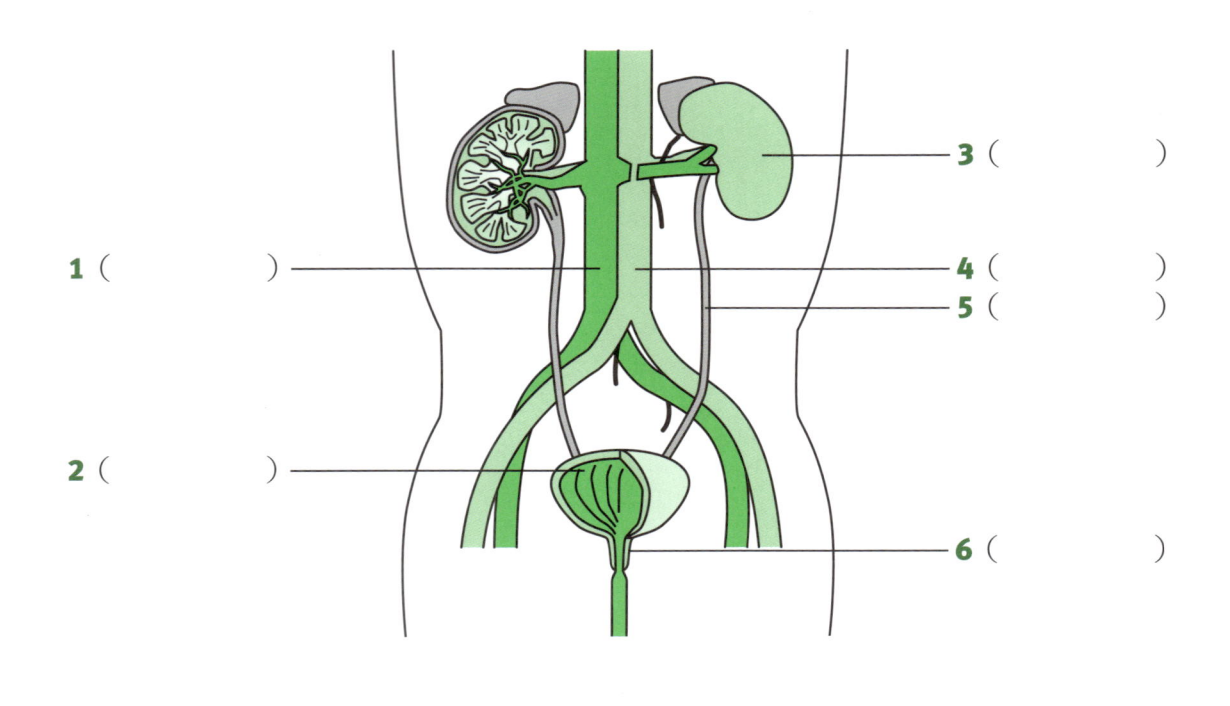

1 (　　　　　)

2 (　　　　　)

3 (　　　　　)

4 (　　　　　)

5 (　　　　　)

6 (　　　　　)

| ⓐ kidney | ⓑ ureter | ⓒ urethra |
| ⓓ inferior vena cava | ⓔ abdominal aorta | ⓕ bladder |

看護師と患者さんの会話を聞いて，以下の質問の答えとして最も適当なものを選びなさい。

1 What is the patient's primary symptom?
- **ⓐ** headache
- **ⓑ** confusion
- **ⓒ** cramps
- **ⓓ** diarrhea

2 What seems to have caused the patient's symptoms?
- **ⓐ** overworking
- **ⓑ** mental stress
- **ⓒ** lack of sleep
- **ⓓ** overeating

3 Why should the patient avoid eating too much meat?
- **ⓐ** It will worsen the kidney.
- **ⓑ** It will worsen the heart.
- **ⓒ** It will worsen the liver.
- **ⓓ** It will worsen the intestines.

4 What other dietary advice is the patient given?
- **ⓐ** Eat more vegetables.
- **ⓑ** Eat less salt.
- **ⓒ** Eat less sugar.
- **ⓓ** Avoid eating spices.

5 How many kilocalories should the patient consume per day?
- **ⓐ** 1,280
- **ⓑ** 1,440
- **ⓒ** 1,600
- **ⓓ** 1,760

Unit 3

Lesson 2

Nurse	Mrs. Spencer, how have you been feeling?
Mrs. Spencer	Well, I've been so busy the last few weeks. And I nearly fell down the other day because I got confused.
Nurse	Do you have any idea what caused the confusion?
Mrs. Spencer	Well, I attended a party at my friend's house, and I may have had too much to eat.
Nurse	Do you have any problems other than the confusion?
Mrs. Spencer	Well, I have had some shortness of breath this week. And I feel like my head has not been clear.
Nurse	You really need to be careful of your diet because what you eat directly affects your condition.
Mrs. Spencer	Yes, I realize that.
Nurse	OK, now let me repeat the instructions given by the doctor. Please avoid eating too much protein. Eating too much meat will produce extra waste in your blood, and that will be a burden on your remaining kidney function.
Mrs. Spencer	Is eating meat twice a week OK?
Nurse	Yes, but it depends on how much you eat. As the dietitian told you before, you do still need to get enough protein. Try eating fish and eggs more often instead.
Mrs. Spencer	OK. I will.
Nurse	And please stick to your low-sodium diet. Use spices to season your food instead of salt.
Mrs. Spencer	Like pepper, ginger, and cloves?
Nurse	Yes, those are especially helpful because they also stimulate your appetite. You are slightly underweight right now, so please be sure to eat 18 units per day. One unit is 80 kilocalories, so that's a total of, let me see... 1,440 kilocalories.
Mrs. Spencer	OK, I understand. I really have to be more careful about my diet.

1 Do you have any idea what caused the confusion?
意識障害になった原因として思い当たることはありますか。

2 Do you have any problems other than the confusion?
意識障害以外に何か問題はありますか。

3 Please avoid eating too much protein.
たんぱく質の摂りすぎは避けてください。

4 Please stick to your low-sodium diet.
低塩食を守ってください。

5 You are slightly underweight right now, so please be sure to eat 18 units per day.
あなたは今，少しやせ気味ですので，1日18ユニットは必ず摂るようにしてください。

Cross-Cultural Topics

世界の臓器移植事情　Organ Transplantation around the World

　1963年，世界で初めての肝臓移植が行われてからこれまでにさまざまな臓器の移植技術が確立されてきています。日本で初めて臓器移植が行われたのは1968年（心臓移植）と比較的早かったものの，当時「脳死は人の死かどうか」をめぐって世論は紛糾しました。移植医療が日本人の伝統的な死生観に抵触したことから移植のための法整備は進まず，多くの患者さんが移植を受けるため海を渡りました。

　2008年の国際移植学会のイスタンブール宣言を受けて，世界保健機関（WHO）は2010年に「必要な臓器は各国内で確保する努力を求める指針」を打ち出したことから日本でも法律が検討され，2010年7月についに改正臓器移植法が施行されました。この法律により「15歳未満からの臓器提供」および「本人の意思が不明な場合は家族の意思による臓器提供」が可能となりました。移植を待つ患者さんが待ち望んだ国内での全年齢での臓器提供の環境が整ったのです。

　しかしながら，日本は現在でも提供数・移植数ともに他の先進諸国に大きな遅れをとっています。2013年度，日本での移植件数は329件だったのに対し，アメリカではその約70倍の22,517件の臓器移植が行われました。その約半数が腎臓単独移植です。

　臓器移植に関する意見は個人によりさまざまです。自分は臓器を提供したいのか，したくないのか，提供するならどの臓器か，提供したくない臓器はあるか等，日頃から臓器移植について考えるとともに，ドナーカードに意思表示をするか，家族と話し合い，自らの意思や家族の意思を確認しておくことが大切です。

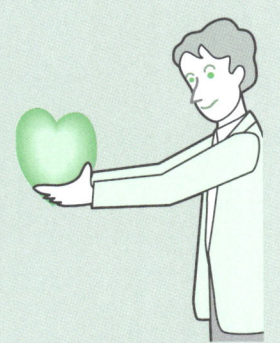

Communication Activity
食事制限についてたずねる Asking about Dietary Restrictions

STEP 1

看護師役と患者さん役に分かれて，以下のモデルダイアローグを練習しましょう。

Example Scenario: Carla Dashan is an Indian engineer. She is a vegetarian because of her religious beliefs. The nurse asks some questions about her dietary restrictions.

Model dialog

Nurse   Mrs. Dashan, do you have any religious restrictions on what you eat?

Mrs. Dashan   Yes, my family strictly adheres to the Hindu religion, so we all avoid eating meat.

Nurse   How about other animal products, such as eggs, cheese, and milk?

Mrs. Dashan   Those are no problem. I often eat them. My aunt is a vegan, but I'm not.

Nurse   All right. Well, do you have any food allergies?

Mrs. Dashan   Not that I know of.

Nurse   OK. If you have any other restrictions on your diet, please let us know.

STEP 2

ボックスの中の表現を使って，以下の会話を練習しましょう。

Scenario 1: Monica Turner comes to the hospital with her son, Willie, a first-grader. Willie presents with symptoms of a severe allergic reaction. He has an allergy to coconut, but he has not had any coconut today. He only drank coffee-flavored milk at school. Mrs. Turner is very worried about him.

Nurse   ① _____

Mrs. Turner   Well, Willie has been suffering from hives and chest pain since he came home from school.

Nurse   ② _____

Mrs. Turner   I'm not sure, but he said he had coffee-flavored milk at school.

Nurse   ③ _____

Mrs. Turner   Really? I didn't know that. I should have advised him to check the ingredients.

Nurse   ④ _____

ⓐ Now, please have Willie lie on the table. The doctor is coming to see him.

ⓑ That's probably the cause. Coconut powder is often added to milk for better taste.

ⓒ OK. What do you think is the cause of his allergic reaction?

ⓓ Mrs. Turner, Willie has a coconut allergy, right? What happened to him?

以下の手順に従って，会話の練習をしましょう。

Scenario 2: Serena Adams is Jewish so her diet is restricted by her religion. Ask her about what she can and cannot eat, especially regarding meat and fish. Then, ask her to fill out a food questionnaire.

Procedure

❶ Greet the patient and ask questions.

❷ Ask the patient whether he/she has any dietary restrictions/allergies.

❸ Ask for further details about the restrictions/allergies. (reasons, symptoms, etc.)

❹ Tell him/her to fill out the questionnaire.

Food Restrictions and Allergies

Judaism (Kosher)
The term Kosher describes all foods permitted for consumption.
• No pork or shellfish.
• Fish is acceptable as long as it has fins and scales.
• Sheep, cows, etc. are allowed.
• Refrain from eating meat and dairy products at the same meal.

Muslims
They have dietary laws called Halaal. During the holy month of Ramadan, Muslims are not allowed to eat from dawn to sunset.
• Carnivorous animals are not permitted.
• All pork and pork products are forbidden.

Hindus and Buddhists
Most Hindus do not eat meat (strict Hindus are vegetarians) and none eat beef since the cow is sacred to them. Strict Buddhists are vegetarians, and their dishes vary since many live in India and China, where available foods will be different.

Vegetarian
Vegetarians are those who do not eat meat or fish, and sometimes other animal products such as eggs and dairy products, especially for moral, religious, or health reasons. Vegans eat only plant foods and products.

Food Allergies
The most common individual food allergies include those to peanuts, tree nuts (walnuts, pecans, etc.), fish, shellfish, eggs, milk, soy, corn, and wheat.

"Food restrictions and allergies." Harvard University Events Managements より引用改変

Other Useful Expressions

Do you have any dietary restrictions?

• I'm on a low-sodium diet.
• I'm diabetic and can only eat 14 units a day.
• I'm Muslim, so I can't eat pork.

Do you have any allergies?

• I'm allergic to milk and cheese.
• I have an allergy to penicillin.
• I have a pollen allergy (hay fever).

Dementia

I Reading and Discussion

以下の文章を読んで患者情報を完成させなさい。また，1～3の質問に英語で答えなさい。

Boris and Andrea Davidson, a couple from Sweden in their mid-sixties, visit the Neurology Department at a university hospital. After Mr. Davidson's retirement from a Swedish-based company last year, they had decided to spend another year in Japan instead of returning to their home country. Having lived in Japan for more than twenty years, Mr. and Mrs. Davidson are not ready to leave yet. Their children, Christina and Peter, are both married and living in Sweden, and they want their parents to come back home so that they can take care of them. However, Mrs. Davidson has recently noticed signs of depression, mild cognitive impairment, and personality change in her husband. Therefore, she worries about their life in Japan and has begun thinking about going back to Sweden. Today she has taken him to the hospital in spite of his reluctance. A nurse asks her several questions about his condition before the doctor's examination.

Patient Information

Name: _____   Nationality: _____

Age: _____   Occupation: _____

Gender: _____   Chief Concerns: _____

Marital Status: _____

1 Why does the patient live in Japan?

2 What is the patient's wife concerned about?

3 What concerns do you think a retired foreign couple living in Japan would have?

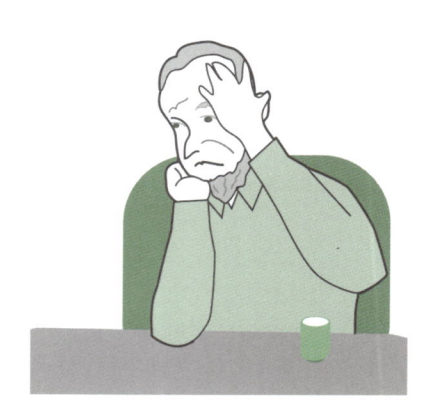

空欄に入る語をボックスから選び，記号で答えなさい。

1 (   ) involves problems with memory, language, or other brain functions.

2 The patient quickly changed between elation and (   ).

3 (   ) includes unusual speech or behavior, anxiety, aggression, etc.

4 (   ) is a chronic disorder of the mental process caused by brain disease or injury.

> **ⓐ** dementia   **ⓑ** depression   **ⓒ** mild cognitive impairment
> **ⓓ** personality change

III **Pre-Listening Vocabulary**

以下の語の定義をボックスから選び，記号で答えなさい。

1 memory loss   (   )

2 irritated   (   )

3 wandering   (   )

4 moody   (   )

> **ⓐ** often unhappy or depressed
> **ⓑ** walking with no direction or purpose
> **ⓒ** not being able to remember new or past events
> **ⓓ** feeling impatient or angry

Unit 3   Lesson 3

IV Extra Vocabulary (Aids for the Elderly)

写真に対応する語をボックスから選び，記号で答えなさい。

1 (　　　　　)

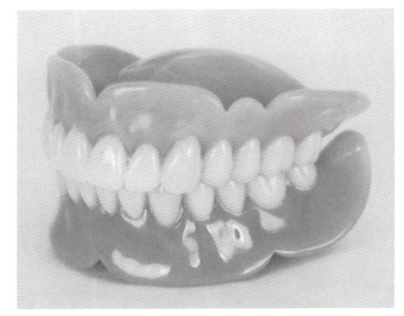

2 (　　　　　)

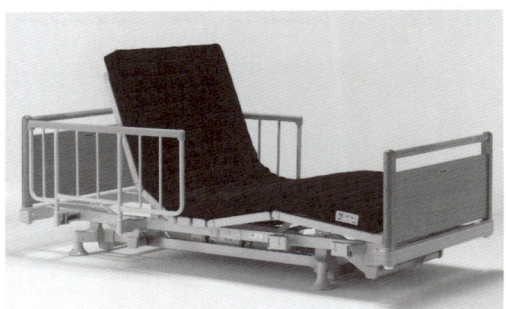

3 (　　　　　)

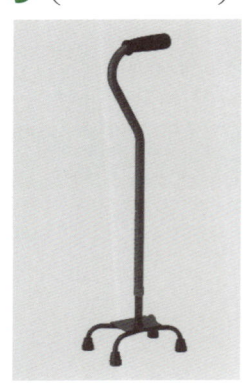

4 (　　　　　)

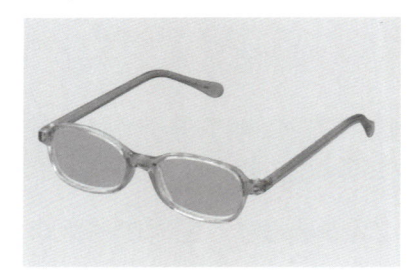

5 (　　　　　)

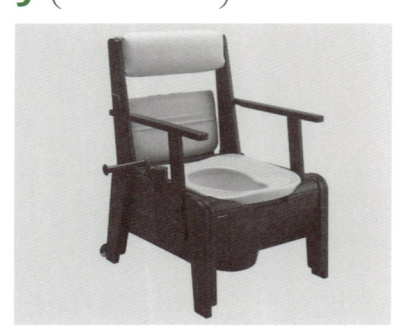

6 (　　　　　)

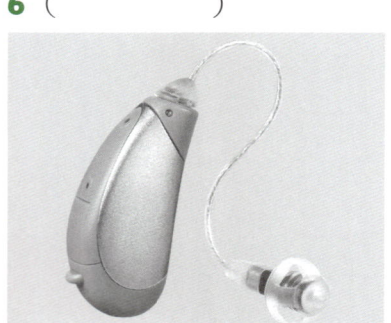

ⓐ dentures　　ⓑ portable toilet　　ⓒ quadruped cane　　ⓓ reclining bed
ⓔ hearing aid　　ⓕ glasses

看護師と患者さんの会話を聞いて，以下の質問の答えとして最も適当なものを選びなさい。

1 What was the first symptom Mrs. Davidson noticed?
- **ⓐ** depression
- **ⓑ** memory loss
- **ⓒ** personality change
- **ⓓ** stress

2 How has the patient's personality changed, according to his wife?
- **ⓐ** He used to be calm, but now he is talkative.
- **ⓑ** He used to be aggressive, but now he is friendly.
- **ⓒ** He used to be shy, but now he is emotional.
- **ⓓ** He used to be active, but now he is unenergetic.

3 When did the patient's symptoms start?
- **ⓐ** last week
- **ⓑ** three weeks ago
- **ⓒ** three months ago
- **ⓓ** last year

4 What does the patient often forget?
- **ⓐ** housework he is supposed to do
- **ⓑ** names of his family and relatives
- **ⓒ** people he is going to meet
- **ⓓ** appointments with doctors

5 Which symptoms does the patient NOT present with?
- **ⓐ** forgetfulness
- **ⓑ** moodiness
- **ⓒ** personality change
- **ⓓ** wandering

Dialog

Nurse	Good morning, Mrs. Davidson. Please tell me about your husband's symptoms.
Mrs. Davidson	Well, I brought Boris today because he seems to have something wrong with him.
Nurse	All right. Can you give me some more details?
Mrs. Davidson	Well, he used to be friendly and kind, and very active on holidays, but lately he rarely goes out. He is moody and gets irritated easily.
Nurse	Oh, really? When did you first notice this change?
Mrs. Davidson	Hmm. I think it was about three months ago.
Nurse	I see. Does he often forget things?
Mrs. Davidson	Yes, quite often these days. He forgets to do little chores around the house that I ask him to do. At first I thought he just didn't want to do them, but now I've begun to realize that he simply doesn't remember.
Nurse	Have you noticed anything else different about him? Like wandering around?
Mrs. Davidson	No, no wandering, but these days he seems sad and stays in his room all day long.
Nurse	So it sounds like he is experiencing personality change, memory loss, and depression.
Mrs. Davidson	Is something wrong with my husband? What should I do for him?
Nurse	You are taking good care of him. The doctor will give you some advice about what you can do for him. Now please wait here for a while.

Key Expressions

1 Can you give me some more details?
もう少し詳しく話していただけませんか。

2 When did you first notice this change?
最初に彼の変化に気付いたのはいつですか。

3 Have you noticed anything else different about him?
他に彼が変わったところはありますか。

4 You are taking good care of him.
よくお世話されていますね。

5 The doctor will give you some advice about what you can do for him.
あなたがご主人にできることについて，医師からアドバイスがあるでしょう。

Cross-Cultural Topics

終の棲家はどこ？ Where is Your Final Home?

　2013年，日本の高齢者（65歳以上）は3,186万人，総人口に占める割合は4人に1人（25％）となり，人数，割合ともに過去最高となりました。この割合は今後も上昇を続け，2035年には33.4％となり，3人に1人が高齢者という超高齢化社会に突入すると推計されています（国立社会保障・人口問題研究所）。現在，高齢者男性の10人に1人，女性の5人に1人が「単身世帯（自宅）」に住んでいますが，老人ホームなどの「施設等」に入居している高齢者の割合は着実に増えつつあります（2010年時点で5.7％）。一方で，国は可能な限り，住み慣れた地域で暮らしたいと願う高齢者のための支援体制の構築にも取り組んでいます。

　福祉大国スウェーデンの高齢者は「終の棲家」をどこに求めているのでしょうか。スウェーデンの高齢者介護政策の原則は「医療や社会的介護を必要とする場合でも高齢者はできるだけ長く自宅で生活を続けること」であり，このために必要な社会サービス（介護手当やバリアフリー化補助金等）が政府によって提供されています。これらのサービスの恩恵により，高齢者の93％が自宅で生活しています。

　2050年には総人口の4人に1人が高齢者となるスウェーデンでは在宅介護を実現する社会保障費と福祉事業費が年々，国家財政を圧迫しています。スウェーデンより早く超高齢化社会に突入するわれわれにとっても他人事ではありません。自宅であれ施設であれ，福祉政策には多大な予算が必要です。減り続ける現役世代の税金だけで高齢者の「終の棲家」を守ることはできるのでしょうか。

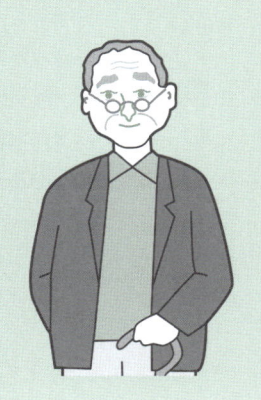

VI Communication Activity
患者の家族を支援する Supporting the Patient's Family

看護師役と患者さん役に分かれて，以下のモデルダイアローグを練習しましょう。

Example Scenario: George Lyman is taking care of his wife, who is bedridden and has dementia. His wife, Mary, hates to wear diapers, so he has to wake up several times every night to assist her in relieving herself. Mr. Lyman feels unwell because of lack of sleep. He has come to the clinic for advice.

Model dialog

Nurse	How is Mary, Mr. Lyman? Is she all right?
Mr. Lyman	Actually she is fine, but I'm not.
Nurse	What's the matter?
Mr. Lyman	She refuses to wear diapers, so she wakes me up every time she needs to go to the toilet.
Nurse	That sounds rough. You will make yourself sick if you continue doing that.
Mr. Lyman	Yes, that's what I'm worried about. I'm really exhausted.
Nurse	You are doing a great job. Let's work together to get some help for Mary.

ボックスの中の表現を使って，以下の会話を練習しましょう。

Scenario 1: Nancy Chopin is depressed because her mother does not remember who she is when she visits her in the hospital. Her mother always says, "How kind of you to visit me here. Can I ask what your name is?" Mrs. Chopin asks the nurse for advice on how to respond when this happens.

Nurse	① _____
Mrs. Chopin	Yes, I want to be with her as much as possible.
Nurse	② _____
Mrs. Chopin	I feel depressed because my mother doesn't recognize me.
Nurse	③ _____
Mrs. Chopin	It's just so shocking every time she does it.
Nurse	④ _____

> ⓐ It's not your fault. That is a common symptom in elderly people.
>
> ⓑ But you look so blue. Are you worried about something?
>
> ⓒ You came to visit your mother again, didn't you?
>
> ⓓ You are doing fine. Now let me give you some tips on how to respond.

以下の手順に従って，会話の練習をしましょう。

Scenario 2: Matthew Keats has been suffering from a lack of appetite. Ever since he had an operation to remove two-thirds of his stomach two months ago, he has had trouble swallowing food because of nausea. His wife, Cecilia, who has come to pick up his medication, is worried about him because he scarcely eats what she cooks for him. Encourage and give advice to Mrs. Keats.

Procedure

❶ Greet the care provider.

❷ Ask the care provider whether he/she has any concerns.

❸ Empathize with the care provider.

❹ Encourage him/her and offer a practical solution if possible.

Other Useful Expressions

1 Do you have any concerns? / Is there anything troubling you?

2 Is there anything I can do for you?

3 You had a hard time, didn't you? But you are doing a great job.

4 I'm afraid I can't. / I wish I could.

5 Let me check with the doctor about that.

6 I'm glad to hear that.

7 Please take good care of yourself.

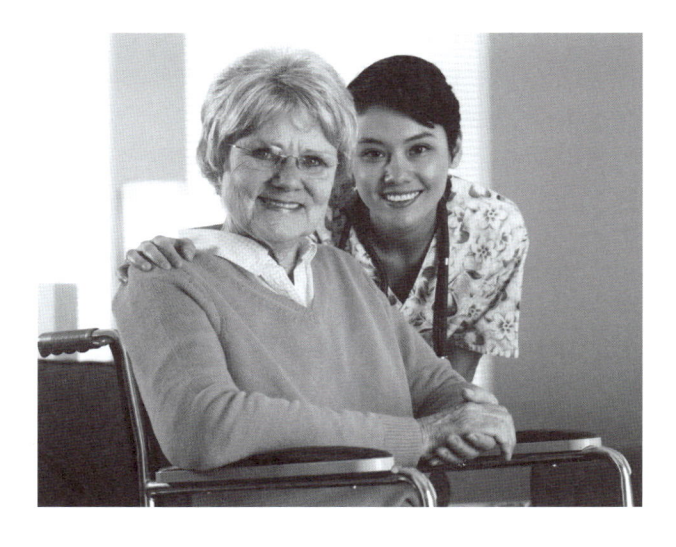

Lifestyle-Related Diseases（生活習慣病）

1	cancer	がん
2	heart disease	心臓病
3	angina pectoris	狭心症
4	stroke	脳卒中
5	myocardial infarction	心筋梗塞
6	diabetes	糖尿病
7	hypertension	高血圧

Others（その他）

1	tumor	腫瘍
2	ulcer	潰瘍
3	bronchitis	気管支炎
4	hepatitis (B)	（B型）肝炎
5	asthma	喘息
6	gout	痛風
7	dementia	認知症
8	depression	うつ病
9	insomnia	不眠症

Infectious Diseases（感染病）

1	measles	麻疹
2	chickenpox	水痘
3	rubella/German measles	風疹
4	mumps	流行性耳下腺炎
5	pertussis/whooping cough	百日咳
6	tetanus	破傷風
7	tuberculosis	結核
8	pneumonia	肺炎

10 Quotes for Student Nurses

1 "To do what nobody else will do, a way that nobody else can do, in spite of all we go through; is to be a nurse." – Rawsi Williams, BSN, RN

2 "They may forget your name but they will never forget how you made them feel." – Maya Angelou

3 "Either you run the day, or the day runs you." – Jim Rohn

4 "Nurses have come a long way in a few short decades. In the past our attention focused on physical, mental and emotional healing. Now we talk of healing your life, healing the environment, and healing the planet." – Lynn Keegan

5 "Behind every great doctor is an even greater nurse." – Unknown

6 "When life puts you in tough situations, don't say 'WHY ME?' Just say 'TRY ME.'" – Unknown

7 "If you wait to do everything until you're sure it's right, you'll probably never do much of anything." – Win Borden

8 "I'm not telling you it's going to be easy, I'm telling you it's going to be worth it." – Arti Williams

9 "Save one life, you're a hero. Save 100 lives, you're a nurse." – Unknown

10 "Nurses are the heart of healthcare." – Donna W. Cardillo

By Pia Love, "10 Motivational Quotes for Student Nurses" © www.NurseTogether.com

Unit 4　入退院ケア

Inpatient Care

　このユニットでは，外来で治療できない病気をかかえ，異文化の中で手術・入院・退院をしなければならない患者さんとその家族のケアについて学びます。厚生労働省によると，2013年の国内における1日平均在院患者数は127万5,347人で，平均在院日数は30.6日でした。病気によって在院日数はさまざまですが，外国人患者さんが入院するということには，手術や治療がうまく行われるかという心配に加えて，病院でいつもの生活が行えるのか，自分の思いや考えを分かってもらえるのかなど，計り知れない不安が伴います。

　ここでは，手術前後のケア，入院中の生活，および退院指導と自宅に戻ってからの在宅ケアについて学びます。医師・看護師・薬剤師・ソーシャルワーカーなどがチームとして協力し，患者さん一人ひとりの状態や希望に沿うことが大切です。

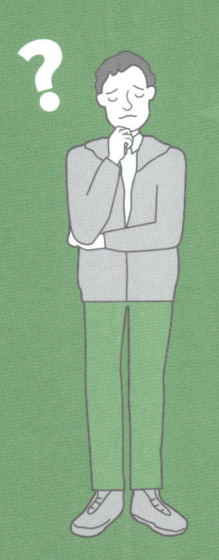

考えてみよう

Q1 昨年医療滞在ビザで入国した
外国人の数はどのくらい？

Q2 イスラム教の患者さんの多くが入院中に
静かな部屋を必要とするのはなぜ？

Q3 全身麻酔を伴う手術後，患者さんは
どのような食事を摂る？

Unit 4 — Lesson 1

Admission for Surgery

I Reading and Discussion

以下の文章を読んで患者情報を完成させなさい。また，1 ～ 3 の設問に英語で答えなさい。

Jack Taylor, a 58-year-old American bank manager, is scheduled for surgery next week. He had pain in the right upper abdomen for two weeks, especially after eating fatty foods such as his favorite fried chicken. He was diagnosed with gallstones and is going to have his gallbladder removed by laparoscopic surgery. The doctor explains to him about the surgery—the procedure (including general anesthesia), the risks, and the need for hospitalization. Mr. Taylor wants to have a day surgery like his friend in the US had. The doctor explains to him that his patients usually stay in the hospital for at least two days after the gallbladder is removed. After some discussion, Mr. Taylor agrees to be hospitalized for two days. The nurse gives him the hospital admission form to fill out and asks if he has someone with him today to be his guarantor, the person responsible for his behavior and payments.

Patient Information

Name: _____ Nationality: _____

Age: _____ Occupation: _____

Gender: _____ Chief Concerns: _____

1 What explanations about the surgery does the doctor give to Mr. Taylor?

2 How long does Mr. Taylor agree to stay in the hospital?

3 What can the nurse do and say to care for a patient who is scheduled for surgery?

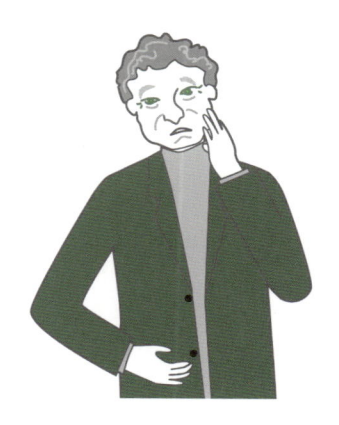

II Post-Reading Vocabulary

空欄に入る語をボックスから選び，記号で答えなさい。

1 My son will be my (   ) and will pay for my expenses if I cannot.

2 In (   ), a surgeon makes small holes instead of one large cut.

3 The nurse arranged the hospital (   ) for the patient.

4 (   ) are formed in the gallbladder, but most people do not know they have them.

ⓐ gallstones	**ⓑ** laparoscopic surgery	**ⓒ** guarantor	**ⓓ** admission

III Pre-Listening Vocabulary

以下の語の定義をボックスから選び，記号で答えなさい。

1 informed consent   (   )

2 urinary catheter   (   )

3 painkiller   (   )

4 inpatient   (   )

> **ⓐ** a thin tube inserted into the body to remove urine from the bladder
>
> **ⓑ** a patient who stays in the hospital and receives treatment
>
> **ⓒ** a patient's formal agreement, after understanding the explanation, to undergo surgery or treatment, or to participate in a clinical study.
>
> **ⓓ** a drug or medicine that relieves pain

写真に対応する語をボックスから選び，記号で答えなさい。

1 (　　　　)

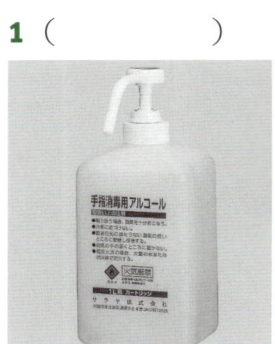

2 (　　　　)

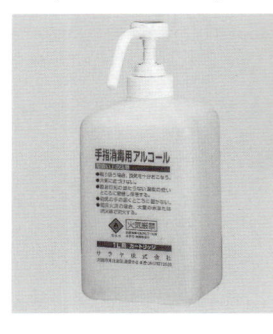

3 (　　　　)

4 (　　　　)

5 (　　　　)

6 (　　　　)

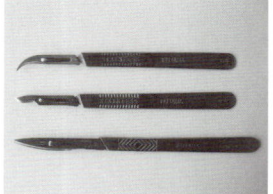

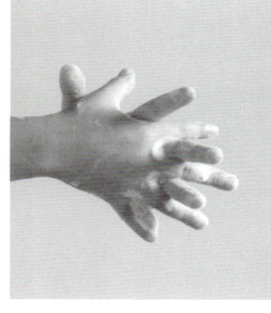

7 (　　　　)

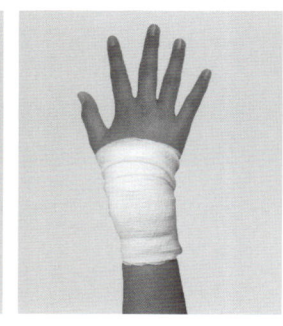

8 (　　　　)

9 (　　　　)

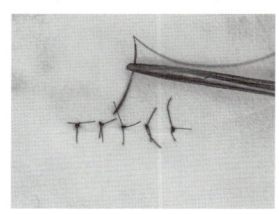

10 (　　　　)

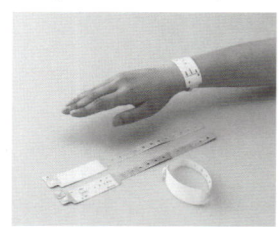

---

a patient ID band	**b** scrubbing	**c** operating room / operating theater
d suture / stitches	**e** scalpel	**f** tweezers / forceps · **g** antiseptic
h vinyl gloves / latex gloves	**i** cotton swab	**j** bandage / dressing

看護師と患者さんの会話を聞いて，以下の質問の答えとして最も適切なものを選びなさい。

1 Who gave Mr. Taylor the informed consent form?
- **ⓐ** his son
- **ⓑ** the nurse
- **ⓒ** the doctor
- **ⓓ** the guarantor

2 Who needs to sign the admission form?
- **ⓐ** only the patient
- **ⓑ** the patient and his wife
- **ⓒ** the patient and his son
- **ⓓ** the patient and the nurse

3 What does the nurse tell Mr. Taylor about the pain?
- **ⓐ** The surgery itself will be painful.
- **ⓑ** He won't have pain during surgery.
- **ⓒ** He won't feel pain at night.
- **ⓓ** The painkillers will not be effective.

4 When will he get his stitches out?
- **ⓐ** He will get them out in a week.
- **ⓑ** He will have them removed in a month.
- **ⓒ** He won't need to have them removed.
- **ⓓ** It depends on when he starts moving around.

5 When will Mr. Taylor be able to move around?
- **ⓐ** the day after the surgery
- **ⓑ** after the IV is taken out
- **ⓒ** when his urinary catheter is removed
- **ⓓ** the following morning

Unit 4

Lesson 1

Nurse   Mr. Taylor, your surgery is scheduled for 9:00 a.m. on May 20th. I think you have already signed the informed consent form with the doctor, right?

Mr. Taylor   Yes, I have.

Nurse   Now, I'd like you to fill out this admission form.

Mr. Taylor   All right. [*He fills out the form and stops.*] I came alone, so I don't have anyone with me who can sign as my guarantor.

Nurse   That's OK. Please do not forget to bring this form with the guarantor's signature on the day of admission.

Mr. Taylor   I'll make sure my son signs it.

Nurse   Do you have any concerns about your surgery?

Mr. Taylor   Is it going to be very painful?

Nurse   Well, you will be under general anesthesia, so you will not feel any pain during the surgery. You might feel some pain as the anesthetic wears off at night, but don't worry, we will do our best to minimize the pain with painkillers. You'll be all right.

Mr. Taylor   When will I get my stitches out?

Nurse   The doctor usually uses stitches that dissolve on their own, so you will probably not need to have them removed.

Mr. Taylor   When will I be able to start moving around?

Nurse   Probably that evening. You will have a urinary catheter inserted into the bladder through the urethra. After we remove that tube, you can walk to the bathroom.

Mr. Taylor   I hope that will be soon.

Nurse   Now, this booklet will tell you about the inpatient facilities and all the information you need during your hospital stay. Please bring your patient ID card, health insurance card, any medicine you are taking, pajamas, a robe, and other items on the list.

1 Your surgery is scheduled for 9:00 a.m. on May 20th.
あなたの手術は 5 月 20 日朝 9 時に予定されています。

2 Please do not forget to bring this form with the guarantor's signature.
保証人が署名したこの書類を忘れないでお持ちください。

3 Do you have any concerns about your surgery?
手術に関してご心配なことは何かありますか。

4 You might feel some pain as the anesthetic wears off.
麻酔が徐々に切れるにしがって少し痛みを感じるかもしれません。

5 You will have a urinary catheter inserted into the bladder.
膀胱には尿道カテーテルが挿入されています。

Cross-Cultural Topics

入院から退院，そして在宅医療へ　From Hospitalization to Home Care

手術の方法，入院日数などは国によって異なり，病院によっても異ります。例えば胆石の腹腔鏡下胆嚢切除術や鼠径ヘルニア手術など，日本でも日帰りで行っている病院もあります。分娩などは，国によっては出産の翌日に退院するところもあれば，1週間入院するところもあります。2013年のOECDの統計によると，普通分娩においてOECD加盟国の平均入院日数は2.9日，イギリスでは1.5日でした。一般に入院日数は日本でも年々減ってきていますが，急性期患者さんの入院平均日数は17.2日と，OECD加盟国の平均8.1日の2倍以上です。さらに，日本は米国などと異なり，急性期だけではなく，回復期の患者さんも入院したまま病棟で治療を受けて退院することが多いので，入院日数は多くなります。

アメリカでは病院は急性期患者さんを診るところで，回復期には退院して，別の施設や自宅で治療を続けます。そしてそのために，入院した時点から，ソーシャルワーカーなどが退院後のサポートの必要性を医療チームと打ち合わせて退院へ向けての準備をしていきます。日本も在宅医療が増えていくなか，入院時からのサポート体制がより充実していくことになるでしょう。

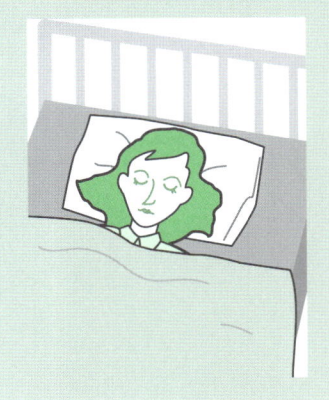

Communication Activity

VI 手術と入院の説明をする Giving Information about Surgery and Hospitalization

STEP 1

看護師役と患者さん役に分かれて，以下のモデルダイアローグを練習しましょう。

Example Scenario: Jane Miller, a 35-year-old Australian, came to the ER with an acute abdominal pain. She was diagnosed with appendicitis and is going to have her appendix removed.

Model dialog

Nurse	Mrs. Miller, is there anything you are concerned about?
Mrs. Miller	What kind of surgery am I going to have? I couldn't catch what the doctor said.
Nurse	You are going to have a laparoscopic surgery, so you may have less pain and a shorter hospital stay.
Mrs. Miller	That's comforting to hear. How long do I have to stay in the hospital?
Nurse	You will probably have to be in hospital for four to five days.
Mrs. Miller	I rushed to the hospital, so I don't have any pajamas or toiletries.
Nurse	That's no problem. You can rent pajamas and buy toiletries here.

STEP 2

ボックスの中の表現を使って，以下の会話を練習しましょう。

Scenario 1: Ann Mason, a 45-year-old American accountant, is having her uterine fibroids removed next month. She is having a hysteroscopic surgery. She is very busy and has a lot of work to finish while she is in the hospital.

Nurse	① _____
Ms. Mason	When will I be able to go home?
Nurse	② _____
Ms. Mason	How much extra do I have to pay to stay in a private room?
Nurse	③ _____
Ms. Mason	I need to work while I'm in the hospital, so I'd like to have a private room.
Nurse	④ _____

ⓐ You will probably be able to go home in one to three days.

ⓑ Do you have any concerns about the surgery?

ⓒ It depends on the availability, but we'll do our best.

ⓓ You need to pay an extra 30,000 yen per day for a private room.

STEP 3

Scenario 2: Charles Jones had been suffering from blurred vision for a long time and has finally decided to have cataract surgery. He is going to have a day surgery. He is concerned about whether it is all right for him to come alone on the day of surgery or not. If not, he wants to know where his wife can wait for him. He also wants to know if he can go to work the next morning after the surgery.

Procedure

❶ Ask whether the patient has concerns about the surgery.

❷ Give information to the patient about the day of surgery.

❸ Give further information about the waiting room.

❹ Give information about the procedure after the surgery and comfort the patient.

Information on Surgeries

The following information may vary depending on the patient's condition.

Surgery	Days of Hospitalization
gallstones	Laparoscopic surgery: 2-3 days Open surgery: 2-3 weeks
appendicitis	Laparoscopic surgery: 4-5 days Open surgery: 7-10 days
uterine fibroids	Hysteroscopic surgery: 1-3 days Laparoscopic surgery: 3-7 days Open surgery: 1-2 weeks
cataract	0*-2 days For day/outpatient surgery, follow-up appointment the next morning

* If you are scheduled for day surgery, please arrange to have someone waiting for you and take you home. You may be feeling sick or dizzy after the surgery. The family waiting area is on the 6th floor.

Information on Admission

* Hospital rooms

Room with 4 beds: no extra charge

Semi-private room with 2 beds: extra 7,500 yen/day

Private room: extra 30,000 yen/day

* List of items to bring

Hospital admission form, health insurance card, patient ID card, medicine, pajamas, towels, nightgown/sweater, toiletries, footwear (not slippers), cup, spoon, chopsticks, etc.

Most items can be bought at the hospital shop on the 1st floor. We also rent out pajamas, gowns, towels, and other items for a fee.

Unit 4

Lesson 1

Daily Life in the Hospital

I Reading and Discussion

以下の文章を読んで患者情報を完成させなさい。また，1 〜 3 の設問に英語で答えなさい。

Hannah Ibrahim, a 47-year-old teacher, has just been hospitalized to have her tonsils removed by surgery tomorrow. The nurse comes in to check her condition. She asks Mrs. Ibrahim how she feels, checks her vital signs—her temperature, pulse, respiratory rate, and blood pressure—and explains to her the daily routine during her stay in the hospital. The nurse also explains to Mrs. Ibrahim all the equipment in the room and the facilities in the ward. Mrs. Ibrahim is a Muslim and has special concerns regarding her religion. She mentioned them when she was filling out the admission form. She is not very worried about the postoperative pain. She is more worried about practicing her religion in the hospital.

Patient Information

Name: _____	Occupation: _____
Age: _____	Chief Concerns
Gender: _____	·Health: _____
Marital Status: _____	·Life in Hospital: _____
Nationality: _____	

1 What does the nurse do in Mrs. Ibrahim's room?

2 What concerns does Mrs. Ibrahim mention when filling out the admission form?

3 What should the nurse know to care for patients from different cultural backgrounds?

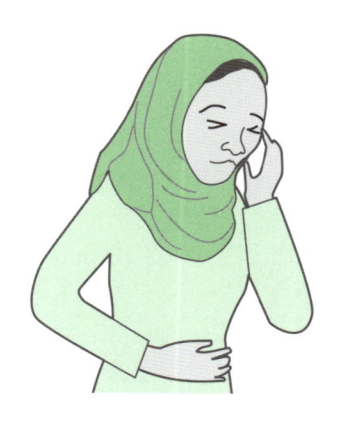

空欄に入る語をボックスから選び，記号で答えなさい。

1 Please be careful not to talk in a loud voice when you are in the hospital
(　　　　　).

2 The patient will be given painkillers for the (　　　　　) pain.

3 It was difficult for her to swallow food because her (　　　　　) were painful.

4 The nurse checked the patient's (　　　　　) to measure her basic bodily functions.

ⓐ vital signs	ⓑ ward	ⓒ tonsils	ⓓ postoperative

Ⅲ Pre-Listening Vocabulary

以下の語の定義をボックスから選び，記号で答えなさい。

1 urination (　　　　　)

2 bowel movement (　　　　　)

3 bed bath (　　　　　)

4 visiting hours (　　　　　)

ⓐ getting rid of waste matter from the large intestine
ⓑ the period of time when family and friends can see a patient in the hospital
ⓒ getting rid of the liquid waste from the bladder
ⓓ washing someone in bed

Unit 4

Lesson 2

写真に対応する語をボックスから選び，記号で答えなさい。

1 (　　　　　)　　2 (　　　　　)　　3 (　　　　　)　　4 (　　　　　)

5 (　　　　　)　　6 (　　　　　)　　7 (　　　　　)　　8 (　　　　　)

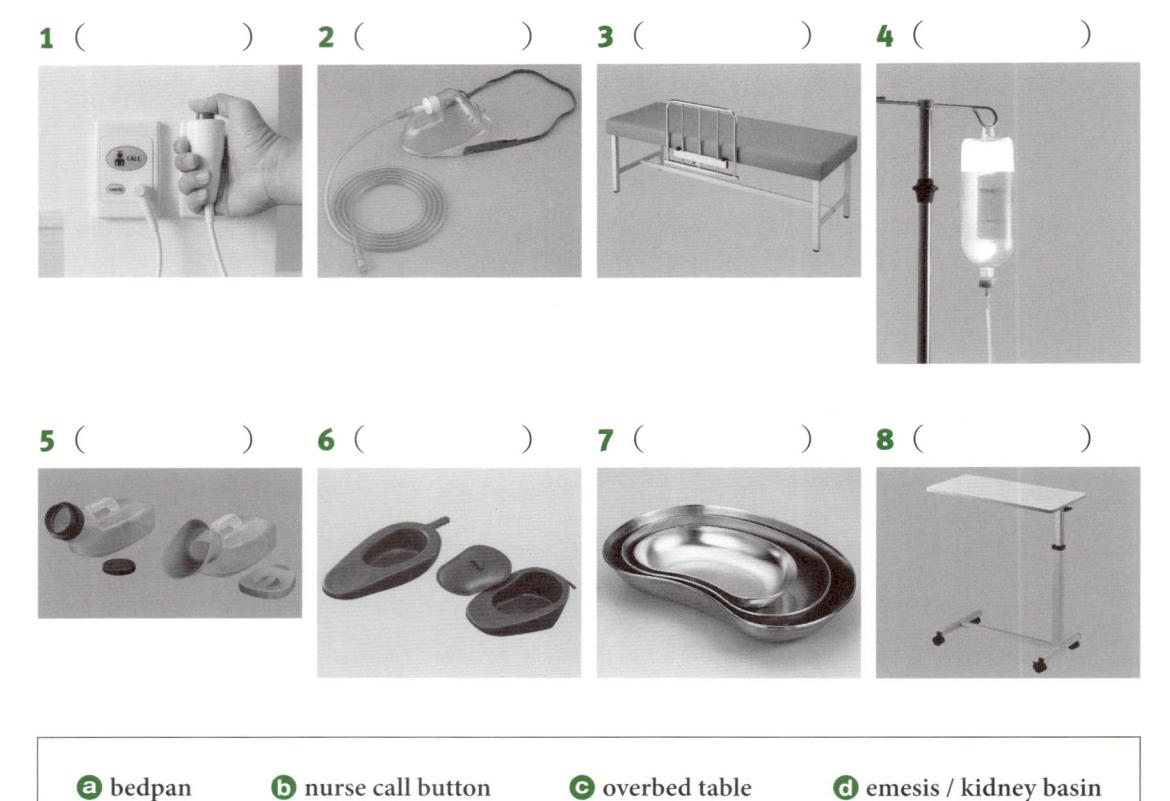

ⓐ bedpan	ⓑ nurse call button	ⓒ overbed table	ⓓ emesis / kidney basin
ⓔ IV drip	ⓕ bedrail	ⓖ oxygen mask	ⓗ urinal

看護師と患者さんの会話を聞いて，以下の質問の答えとして最も適当なものを選びなさい。

1 What does the nurse NOT do every morning?
- ⓐ take the patient's blood pressure
- ⓑ take a blood sample
- ⓒ ask about bowel movements and urination
- ⓓ take the patient's temperature

2 What does the nurse tell Mrs. Ibrahim about her meals?
- ⓐ She can have an ordinary breakfast tomorrow.
- ⓑ She cannot eat or drink anything today.
- ⓒ She is on a liquid diet until 9:00 p.m. tonight.
- ⓓ She can eat until 9:00 p.m. tonight.

3 Where can Mrs. Ibrahim use her mobile phone?
- ⓐ anywhere in the hallway
- ⓑ in the special area
- ⓒ near the elevators
- ⓓ where the payphones are

4 What does the nurse say Mrs. Ibrahim can do after the surgery tomorrow?
- ⓐ She can have a bed bath.
- ⓑ She can take a shower.
- ⓒ She can take a bath.
- ⓓ She can have a foot bath.

5 What concern does Mrs. Ibrahim mention regarding her religion?
- ⓐ She cannot eat pork.
- ⓑ She has to have the lights turned off at 8:00 p.m.
- ⓒ She cannot take certain medicine.
- ⓓ She wants a private space so that she can pray.

Nurse	Good afternoon, Mrs. Ibrahim. Have you settled down in your room?
Mrs. Ibrahim	Yes, thank you.
Nurse	Your surgery is at 10:00 tomorrow morning. How are you feeling?
Mrs. Ibrahim	Nervous.
Nurse	You'll be fine. Now, I'd like to explain to you the daily routine in the hospital.
Mrs. Ibrahim	All right.
Nurse	Every morning, a nurse will come to take your temperature and blood pressure and ask you about your urination and bowel movements. Breakfast is from 7:30, but I'm afraid you will not be able to eat breakfast tomorrow.
Mrs. Ibrahim	That's too bad.
Nurse	I'm sorry…Please do not eat anything after 9:00 tonight.
Mrs. Ibrahim	All right. [*With her mobile phone in hand*] My husband wants to come now. Is that all right?
Nurse	The visiting hours are from 2:00 to 8:00 p.m., so he should come a little later. Also, please use your mobile phone in the special area at the end of the hallway.
Mrs. Ibrahim	OK. I will just text him then. Can I take a shower now?
Nurse	Well, you need to reserve the shower room first. I'll check what time you can use the shower.
Mrs. Ibrahim	I guess I won't be able to take a shower after the surgery tomorrow, right?
Nurse	Well, you won't be able to take a shower tomorrow, but I can give you a bed bath.
Mrs. Ibrahim	Oh, that would be nice.
Nurse	Do you have any questions or concerns regarding your religion or anything else?
Mrs. Ibrahim	Well, I mentioned this before admission, but I would like to have a quiet place where I can pray.
Nurse	Yes. As you have told us in advance, we were able to get a small room for you. If you have any other concerns, just press the nurse call button anytime.

1 I'd like to explain to you the daily routine in the hospital.
入院中の日課をご説明します。

2 Every morning, a nurse will come to take your temperature.
毎朝，看護師が体温を測りにきます。

3 Please use your mobile phone in the special area.
携帯電話は決められた場所でお使いください。

4 I can give you a bed bath.
ベッドの上で体をお拭きできますよ。

5 Just press the nurse call button anytime.
いつでもナースコールボタンを押してください。

Cross-Cultural Topics

入院生活を支えるケア　Supporting Patients' Daily Life in the Hospital

　入院中は，病気のケアはもちろんのこと，心のケア，そして患者さんにとっては今まで当たり前だった日常の生活が尊重されるようなケアが必要となります。

　さまざまな宗教の信者にとって「祈り」は生活の一部であり，入院中も行えるような配慮が大切です。イスラム教徒は，メッカの方に向かって1日に5回礼拝を行います。カトリック信者も日々の祈りを大切にし，手術前には司祭や家族・友人が集まり，共に祈りを捧げる人も多くいます。

　食事では，甲殻類アレルギーの人には，料理にそのエキスが入っていないか，豚肉を食べないイスラム教徒の食事にはブイヨンやゼラチンなども入っていないかなど細かい注意が必要となります。薬を服用する際も，冷水ではなくお湯を好む文化もあります。

　入院中の看護に関しては，日本の病院の多くは完全看護ですが，家族が24時間患者さんに付き添うことを当然とし，夜も付き添いを希望する外国人家族もいます。このような希望については，入院が決まった時点で患者さんとよく話し合い，病院ができることとできないこと，ルール等を明らかにしながら解決策を探していくことが大切でしょう。

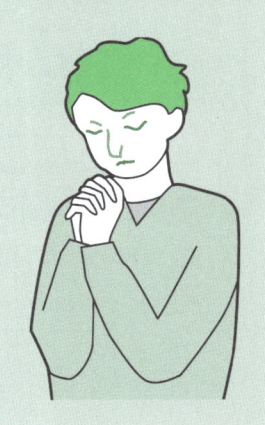

Communication Activity
入院中の生活を補助する Helping Patients during Their Hospital Stay

STEP 1

看護師役と患者さん役に分かれて，以下のモデルダイアローグを練習しましょう。

Example Scenario: Sarah Thomson, a 62-year-old Catholic from Australia, is having a heart surgery in two days. Her priest and the whole family are coming to her bedside to pray for her at noon tomorrow. Mrs. Thomson is in a six-bed room. It is already 8:00 in the evening. She calls the nurse.

Model dialog

Nurse	Mrs. Thomson, what can I do for you?
Mrs. Thomson	My priest and my family want to come tomorrow at noon to pray for me.
Nurse	The visiting hours are from 2:00 to 8:00 p.m. Can they come during the visiting hours?
Mrs. Thomson	No. My priest can only come at that time.
Nurse	Well, let me find a private room for you.
Mrs. Thomson	Thank you very much. Can I take a shower first thing tomorrow morning?
Nurse	I will book a time for you, and hand over your request to the nurse in the morning.

STEP 2

ボックスの中の表現を使って，以下の会話を練習しましょう。

Scenario 1: Isabella Mills is 84 years old. She wants to go home for the weekend because her grandson is coming home from India. She needs the doctor's permission to stay home overnight. She calls the nurse.

Nurse	① _____
Mrs. Mills	I want to go home for the weekend.
Nurse	② _____
Mrs. Mills	When is he coming in?
Nurse	③ _____
Mrs. Mills	Could you tell him when he comes in?
Nurse	④ _____
Mrs. Mills	Thank you very much.

ⓐ I am leaving soon at 8:00 this morning, so I will pass on your request to the other nurses.

ⓑ I think it will be all right, but you need to ask your doctor for permission.

ⓒ Good morning, Mrs. Mills. How can I help you?

ⓓ I'm not quite sure. He usually drops by at the nurses' station around 9:30 a.m.

以下の手順に従って，会話の練習をしましょう。

Scenario 2: Peter Tabak, a 20-year-old Canadian university student, has broken his leg and is staying in the hospital. He wants to use the Internet every day to write his paper. However, he is in a four-bed room and he cannot get connected. He calls the nurse.

Procedure

❶ Greet the patient and listen to the patient's request.

❷ Tell the patient about the facilities in the hospital.

❸ Try to help the patient.

❹ Assure the patient that you will hand off (hand over) the patient's request to the other nurses.

Daily Routine	
7:00 a.m.	Nurse checks condition (temperature/pulse/blood pressure/urination/bowel movements)
7:30 a.m.	Breakfast (liquid diet/pureed foods/soft foods/regular meal)
8:30 a.m.	Doctor's rounds Please stay in your room.
11:30 a.m.	Lunch
3:00 p.m.	Nurse checks temperature/pulse/blood pressure
6:00 p.m.	Dinner
7:30 p.m.	Nurse checks temperature/pulse/blood pressure
9:00 p.m.	Lights go off

* Please wear your patient ID band at all times.

* Shower: 10:00 a.m. – 7:00 p.m.
　　　　(Please check with the doctor and reserve the time with the nurse.)
* The TV and washing machine can be used by buying a pre-paid card.
* Wireless Internet access is available in the dayroom and private rooms.
* Visiting hours: 2:00-8:00 p.m.
* Doctor's permission is needed for going out of the hospital or staying overnight.

Other Useful Expressions

1 Yes. Let me find out what time you can use the shower room.

2 Let me check that with the doctor.

3 You need to check that with the doctor.

4 I will let the other nurses know.

5 I will hand over your request to the nurses on the next shift.

Lesson 3
Discharge and Home Care

I Reading and Discussion

以下の文章を読んで患者情報を完成させなさい。また，1 〜 3 の設問に英語で答えなさい。

Tony Chan, a 75-year-old man, is suffering from lung cancer. He had a small part of his lung removed eight days ago. After the surgery, he had a chest tube placed into his lung and was put on oxygen. Now that everything has been removed, he is going to be discharged tomorrow. The nurse comes in to arrange the discharge. She is in charge of explaining the details of home care. She asks Mr. Chan a couple of questions but then goes back to the nurses' station to wait for his son to arrive. The nurse wants to go over the discharge instructions with his family present as they are the ones who are going to take care of him at home. Mr. Chan's wife is already in his room, but she only speaks Chinese. The nurse also knows that Mr. Chan prefers his son to be in charge of everything at home. The son arrives, and the nurse explains to the family about home care—particularly wound care and medication. Mr. Chan's next appointment is on January 8th. After careful examination, the doctor will decide when to start oral chemotherapy and prescribe medicine to be taken home.

Patient Information

Name: _____	Marital Status: _____
Age: _____	Nationality: _____
Gender: _____	Chief Concerns: _____

1 Who does the nurse want to talk with about home care?

2 When will Mr. Chan learn the details of his oral chemotherapy?

3 What other information on home care do you think a nurse needs to give to a patient?

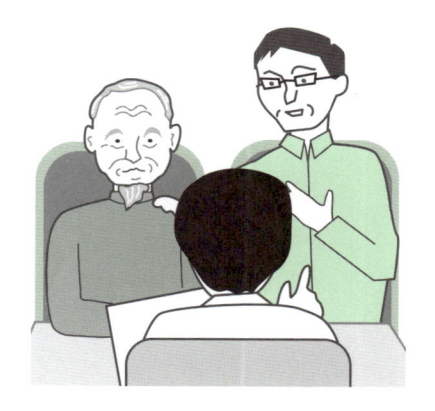

II Post-Reading Vocabulary

空欄に入る語をボックスから選び，記号で答えなさい。

1 He is taking (　　　　　) to treat his cancer.

2 The patient had a (　　　　　) inserted to remove blood.

3 After (　　　　　), the patient's wife has to take care of the patient at home.

4 Proper (　　　　　) is important to avoid infection and help the healing process.

ⓐ chest tube	ⓑ discharge	ⓒ wound care	ⓓ oral chemotherapy

III Pre-Listening Vocabulary

以下の語の定義をボックスから選び，記号で答えなさい。

1 drowsiness　　　　　(　　　　　)

2 general practitioner (GP)　(　　　　　)

3 home care　　　　　(　　　　　)

4 caregiver　　　　　(　　　　　)

ⓐ a person who helps someone who cannot take care of himself/herself

ⓑ sleepiness

ⓒ a physician who provides primary health care to patients of all ages

ⓓ care provided to a patient where he/she lives

IV Extra Vocabulary (Respiratory System)

イラストに対応する語をボックスから選び，記号で答えなさい。

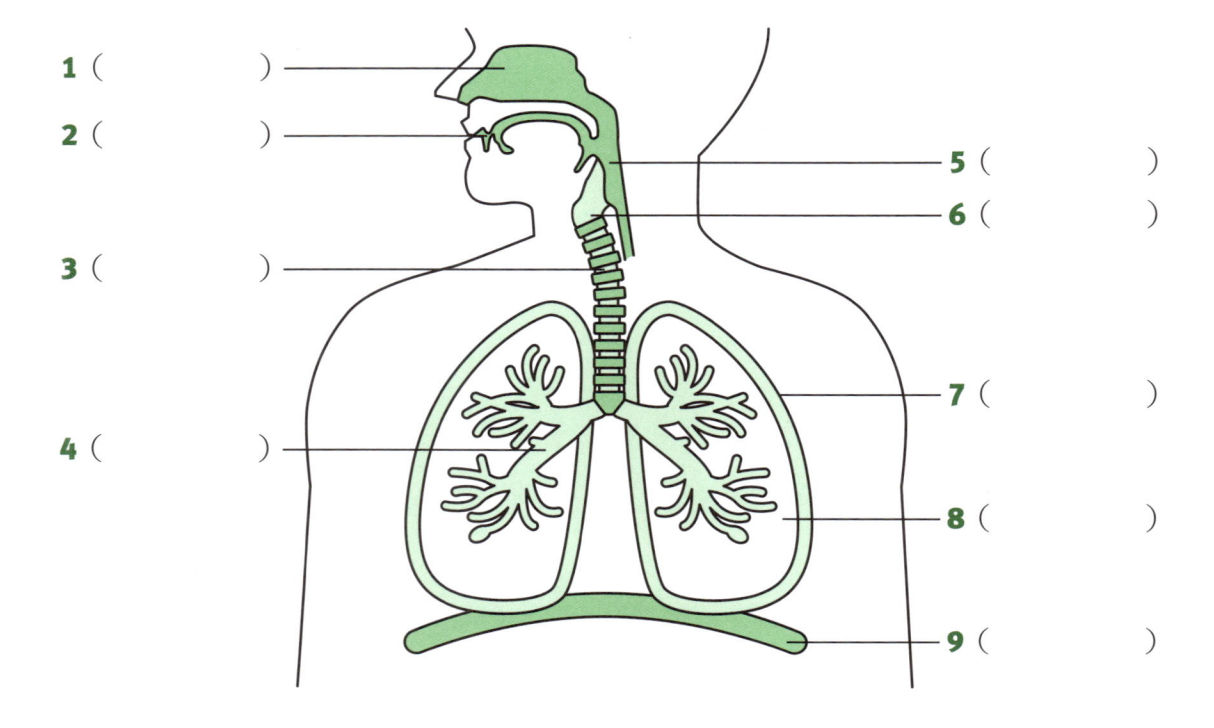

1 (　　　　　)

2 (　　　　　)

3 (　　　　　)

4 (　　　　　)

5 (　　　　　)

6 (　　　　　)

7 (　　　　　)

8 (　　　　　)

9 (　　　　　)

ⓐ diaphragm　　ⓑ bronchus　　ⓒ trachea　　ⓓ larynx　　ⓔ pharynx　　ⓕ pleura
ⓖ nasal cavity　　ⓗ lung　　ⓘ oral cavity

看護師と患者さんの会話を聞いて，以下の質問の答えとして最も適当なものを選びなさい。

1 What did the nurse bring to Mr. Chan with his medicine?
- **ⓐ** warm tea
- **ⓑ** warm water
- **ⓒ** cold water
- **ⓓ** grapefruit juice

2 What does the family have to do first thing tomorrow morning?
- **ⓐ** come upstairs to pay the bill
- **ⓑ** go to the first floor to get medicine
- **ⓒ** come upstairs to hear about discharge procedures
- **ⓓ** go to the first floor to the cashier

3 What side effects might Mr. Chan get from the medicine he is taking home tomorrow?
- **ⓐ** chest pain
- **ⓑ** loss of hair
- **ⓒ** nausea
- **ⓓ** shortness of breath

4 Who helped the nurse find Ms. Mariko Nakagawa?
- **ⓐ** the caregiver
- **ⓑ** Mr. Chan's son
- **ⓒ** the social worker
- **ⓓ** the pharmacist

5 What should Mr. Chan do at home?
- **ⓐ** start chemotherapy
- **ⓑ** take a warm bath
- **ⓒ** get enough rest
- **ⓓ** wash and scrub the wound

Unit 4

Lesson 3

Nurse   How are you feeling, Mr. Chan? Here's your medicine with some warm water.

Mr. Chan   Thank you very much. I prefer warm water.

Nurse   Since your son is with us now, I'd like to explain to you the discharge procedure and home care. Please stop me anytime if you have any questions.

Mr. Chan   Thank you.

Nurse   First thing tomorrow morning, please go to the cashier on the first floor and settle the payment. Then come back upstairs, and the pharmacist will give you the medicines to take home. You may get slight side effects such as nausea or drowsiness.

Mr. Chan   When will I start oral chemotherapy?

Nurse   The doctor will decide that after your next visit.

Mr. Chan   All right.

Nurse   We have coordinated your home care with the social worker. A caregiver, Mariko Nakagawa, will come every day to help you.

Mr. Chan   Thank you very much. I am relieved to hear that.

Nurse   Mr. Chan, please see your GP regularly and take it easy at home. Rest as much as you can—you'll get tired easily.

Mr. Chan   Can I take a shower?

Nurse   You can take a quick shower, but do not scrub the wound. Dry the area around your wound with a clean cloth and change the bandage.

1 I'd like to explain to you the discharge procedure and home care.
退院と自宅でのケアについて説明したいと思います。

2 Please go to the cashier on the first floor and settle the payment.
1階の会計に行って支払いを済ませてください。

3 You may get slight side effects such as nausea or drowsiness.
吐き気や眠気などの副作用が少しあるかもしれません。

4 We have coordinated your home care with the social worker.
あなたの在宅ケアをソーシャルワーカーとコーディネートしました。

5 Please see your GP regularly and take it easy at home.
かかりつけ医に定期的に診てもらい，家で静養してください。

Cross-Cultural Topics

一人ひとりの最期の時　A Person's Last Moment

　最期の時の迎え方は文化によって，宗教によって，そして人によってさまざまです。それは時代とともに変化します。

　欧米では，患者さんが自分らしく生き，自分の望む人生を終えるためには，どのような治療や介護を受け，どこでどのように人生の終わりを迎えたいのかの意思表明を残すリビング・ウィルが一般的になっています。さらに，自ら意思表示ができなくなったときにはその思いを誰に託すのか，医療判断代理委任状を残すこともあります。医療判断代理人は患者さんのケアに携わる医療者ではなく，患者さんが信頼でき，患者さんとよく話し合い，患者さんの望みを代弁できる人です。患者さんの意思を示した書類は，経年的な気持ちの変化にも対応できるよう見直されていきます。国によって法的拘束力のあるものとないものがありますが，人生の最終段階で「望ましい死」について考え，できるだけ患者さんの望みに寄り添ったケアが行われているのです。

　日本においても，患者さんがどのように生きて，よりよく人生を終わりたいかという患者さんの意思を表現できる体制をさらに整えていくことが必要でしょう。日本では，患者さんの意思もさることながら，医療者との関係，家族との関係や家族の意向が重視されたりすることもあります。リビング・ウィルは，日本の文化や家族関係に合わせて発展させることで，より一般的になり，その人らしい生き方を支援するケアにつながっていくでしょう。

　宗教によっては終わりを迎える前に伝統的な儀式を行います。欧米の病院に限らず，アジア・中東などの病院にもChaplainがいて，死を待つ患者さんの部屋を訪ねて静かに話を聞いたり，一緒に祈りを捧げたりします。患者さんの信仰する個別の宗教の聖職者が病室を訪ねることもあります。キリスト教のカトリック信者は，司祭（神父）が立ち会い，「病者の塗油の秘跡」を授けてもらいます。患者さんは最期の祈りを捧げ，家族は患者さんの死後も祈りを捧げます。同じ宗教を信じる人たちの間でも望みが異ることもあります。異文化を理解する際には，固定観念で判断してしまうことなく，一人ひとりと真摯に向き合って寄り添っていくことが大切でしょう。

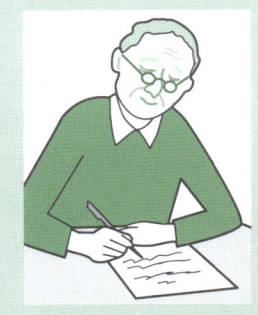

Communication Activity

退院指導をする Giving Discharge Instructions

STEP 1

看護師役と患者さん役に分かれて，以下のモデルダイアローグを練習しましょう。

Example Scenario: Timothy Brown, an 87-year-old man from England, is going to be discharged today. He is given information on his medication, but he does not like the powdered medicine.

Model dialog

Nurse　　Mr. Brown, don't forget to take the medicine after every meal, three times a day.

Mr. Brown　Yes, but I don't like this powdered medicine in sachets. We never have this kind of medicine in our country, and it's so difficult to swallow.

Nurse　　I understand, but please drink some water and take it as directed.

Mr. Brown　All right. The good thing is that it does not have any side effects.

Nurse　　I'm glad to hear that. Now, your next appointment is on September 10th at 9:00 a.m.

Mr. Brown　Yes, next month. How will I know if I should call the hospital immediately?

Nurse　　If the pain gets worse, call the hospital and come as soon as possible.

Mr. Brown　I hope that won't happen.

STEP 2

ボックスの中の表現を使って，以下の会話を練習しましょう。

Scenario 1: Raoul Parma, a 69-year-old Italian, is going to be discharged today. He tells the nurse that he gets nauseated from the side effects of the medicine. He is worried because he lives alone.

Nurse　　① _____

Mr. Parma　I will, but I feel a bit sick when I take this medicine.

Nurse　　② _____

Mr. Parma　Just a little. I guess it's all right.

Nurse　　Let me know if it gets worse.　③ _____

Mr. Parma　Yes, at 10:00. I'm worried about my condition. How will I know if I should rush to the hospital?

Nurse　　④ _____

Mr. Parma　I hope I'll be all right.

ⓐ Now, your next visit to the hospital is scheduled for 10:00 a.m. on May 22nd.

ⓑ Come to the hospital immediately if you develop chest pain and shortness of breath.

ⓒ Mr. Parma, please be sure to take this medicine, one pill after each meal.

ⓓ Some people do get nauseated from this medicine. Do you feel very sick?

以下の手順に従って，会話の練習をしましょう。

Scenario 2: Charlotte Kang is an 81-year-old Korean. The hospital has arranged her discharge with her family and her caregiver. Mrs. Kang does not like the medicine she is taking. The capsule is huge and it is very difficult for her to swallow. It sticks in her throat. Her next appointment is on December 20th at 1:00 p.m.

Procedure

❶ Give instructions for medication.

❷ Understand the patient's concern about the medicine and give advice.

❸ Confirm the next appointment.

❹ Give instructions on emergency situations (when to call the hospital or 119).

Discharge Instructions		
Patient	Raoul Parma (69 years old)	Charlotte Kang (81 years old)
GP	Dr. Tony Sasaki Tel: 5090-2130	Dr. Catherine Wilson Tel: 5090-7856
Support at home	Caregiver: Takeshi Nakano Tel: 2257-3310	Caregiver: Yuko Kaneda Tel: 5081-4622 Daughter and daughter-in-law take turns staying overnight.
Activities	Rest needed	Complete rest needed Needs help in most activities. (Dressing, going to the bathroom, etc.)
Wound care	Shower with soap and water (No bath until doctor's permission) Change bandage.	Keep the area clean and dry. No showers. If the dressing gets wet, remove it, and replace with a dry dressing.
Medication	1 pill after meals Possible side effect: nausea	2 capsules every 6 hours No side effects reported
Next appointment	May 22nd at 10:00 a.m.	December 20th at 1:00 p.m.
Call the hospital or 119 immediately	If you get chest pain and shortness of breath	If you develop a high fever

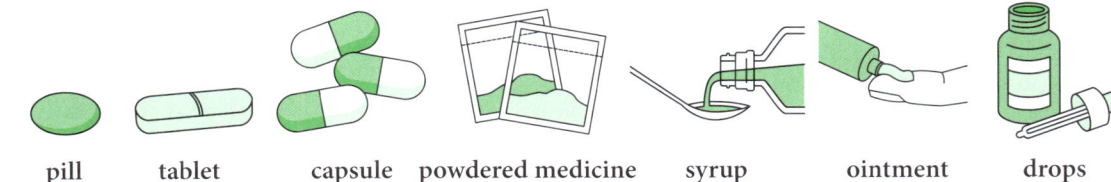

pill   tablet   capsule   powdered medicine   syrup   ointment   drops

Remember the "five rights."

1 the right patient   3 the right time   5 the right route

2 the right drug   4 the right dose

Measurements and Tests（計測と検査）

1	計測	**body measurement**
	身長	**height**
	体重	**weight**
2	体脂肪率	**body mass index (BMI)**
3	血圧（*blood pressure gauge; sphygmomanometer* 血圧計）	**blood pressure**
4	心拍数	**heart rate**
5	呼吸数	**respiratory rate**
6	脈拍	**pulse**
7	体温（*thermometer* 体温計）	**temperature**
8	肺の検査（*stethoscope* 聴診器）	**lung exam**
9	頭頸部検査（*tongue depressor* 舌圧子；患者の舌を押さえるもの）	**head and neck exam**
10	神経学的検査（*reflex hammer* 打診器・打腱器）	**neurological exam**
11	尿検査	**urine test (urinalysis)**
12	血液検査	**blood test (hemanalysis)**
13	検便	**stool test**
14	喀痰検査	**sputum test**
15	胸部 X 線検査	**chest X-ray**
16	肺機能検査（*spirometer* 肺活量計）	**spirometry**
17	心電図検査	**electrocardiography (ECG/EKG)**
18	腹部超音波検査	**abdominal ultrasonography**
19	聴力検査（*otoscope* 耳鏡）	**hearing test (hearing acuity test)**
20	眼の検査（*ophthalmoscope* 検眼鏡）	**eye test**
	視力検査	**eyesight test (visual acuity test)**
	眼圧検査	**eye pressure test**
	眼底検査	**fundus examination**
21	コンピューター断層撮影	**computed tomography (CT)**
22	磁気共鳴断層撮影	**magnetic resonance imaging (MRI)**
23	脳波検査	**electroencephalography (EEG)**
24	陽電子放射断層撮影	**positron emission tomography (PET)**
25	胃腸内視鏡検査	**gastrointestinal endoscopy**
26	大腸内視鏡検査	**colonoscopy**
27	乳房レントゲン撮影法	**mammography**
28	生体組織検査（生検）	**biopsy**

Glossary

A

acute　急性の
aggression　攻撃性
anxiety　不安，恐れ
as directed　指示通り
aspirin　アスピリン
attend to　～に反応する

B

be diagnosed with　～と診断される
bedridden　寝たきりの
bleeding　出血
blockage　妨害物
blood loss　分娩後の出血
blood sample　血液サンプル
blurred vision　かすみ目，視覚低下
breastfeed　授乳する
burn　やけど（する）

C

carnivorous　肉食の
cataract　白内障
Celsius　摂氏
choke　詰まらせる
clinical study　臨床研究
constipation　便秘
crown　胎児の頭が出てくる
cuff　カフ，加圧帯

D

daily routine　日課
day/outpatient surgery　日帰り手術
diabetic　糖尿病患者
diaper　おむつ
diarrhea　下痢
dissolve　溶ける
dizzy　目まいがする
doctor's rounds　医者の回診

E

elation　高揚
exhausted　疲労困憊した

F

Fahrenheit　華氏
fill out　記入する
first trimester　妊娠初期
flex　曲げる
fluids　水分
foot bath　足浴

G

gestational diabetes　妊娠糖尿病
gown　病衣

H

hand over (hand off)　後任に引き渡す
hives　蕁麻疹

hospital admission form　入院手続き
　書類

hurt　痛む

hysteroscopic surgery　子宮鏡下手術

I

immune system　免疫システム

impurities　不純物

infection　感染

influenza/flu　インフルエンザ

ingredient　材料

inhale　息を吸う

insomnia　不眠症

irregular　不規則な

L

labor　陣痛，分娩

lack of appetite　食欲不振

liquid diet　流動食

lower back pain　腰痛

lukewarm　ぬるい

lung cancer　肺がん

M

make a fist　こぶしを握る

menopause　閉経，更年期

menorrhagia　月経過多（症）

menstrual cycle　月経周期

menstrual pain　月経痛

minimize　最小限にする

morning sickness　つわり

Mother and Child Health Handbook
　母子手帳

N

nausea　嘔気

nauseated　吐き気がする

nurses' station　ナースステーション

O

OB/GYN　産婦人科

on duty　勤務中の

open surgery　開腹手術

overreaction　過剰反応

oxygen　酸素

P

painless　痛くない

pain medicine/medication　鎮痛剤

pelvic exam　内診

persistently　永続的な, ひっきりなしに
　繰り返される

placenta　胎盤

pregnancy test　妊娠検査

pregnant　妊娠した

prick　ちくっとすること

pulse　脈拍

pulse oximeter　パルスオキシメーター

pureed food　裏ごしされた食べ物

push　いきむ

R

rash　発疹

redness　発赤

reimburse　費用を払い戻す

relieve　緩和する，和らげる

reroute　〜を迂回させる

running water　流水

runny nose　鼻水

S

sachet　小袋

scar　傷跡，ケロイド

screening　スクリーニング

social worker　ソーシャルワーカー，社会福祉士

solid food　固形食

stroke　脳卒中

suffer from　〜を患う

surgical incision　外科的切開

swallow　飲み込む，嚥下する

T

teething　生歯

throbbing　ずきずきする

tingling　チクチクする痛み

tissue　組織

toiletries　洗面用具

tourniquet　止血帯

type 2 diabetes　2型糖尿病

U

ulcer　潰瘍

unenergetic　活力のない

urine sample　尿の検体

uterine fibroid　子宮筋腫

V

vegan　完全菜食主義者

vegetarian　菜食主義者

vomit　吐く

W

waste　排泄物

weaning　離乳

wear off　効果が徐々に消えていく

weight gain　体重増加

whiplash　むち打ち

worsen　悪化させる

すぐに使える医療・看護英語
English for Healthcare Communication

2016年1月10日　第1版第1刷発行
2019年3月10日　　　第3刷発行

■著　者　井上麻未，松岡里枝子，芦田ルリ，
　　　　　宮津多美子，Jeffrey Huffman

■発行者　三澤　岳

■発行所　株式会社メジカルビュー社
　　　　　〒162-0845 東京都新宿区市谷本村町2-30
　　　　　電話　03(5228)2050(代表)
　　　　　ホームページ http://www.medicalview.co.jp/

　　　　　営業部　FAX 03(5228)2059
　　　　　　　　　E-mail eigyo@medicalview.co.jp

　　　　　編集部　FAX 03(5228)2062
　　　　　　　　　E-mail ed@medicalview.co.jp

■印刷所　シナノ印刷株式会社

ISBN978-4-7583-0759-8 C3047

©MEDICAL VIEW, 2016.　Printed in Japan